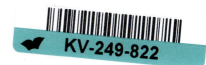

on   020 7   /449

                    c.uk

The Family Therapy Collections

James C. Hansen, Series Editor

Marion Lindblad-Goldberg, Volume Editor

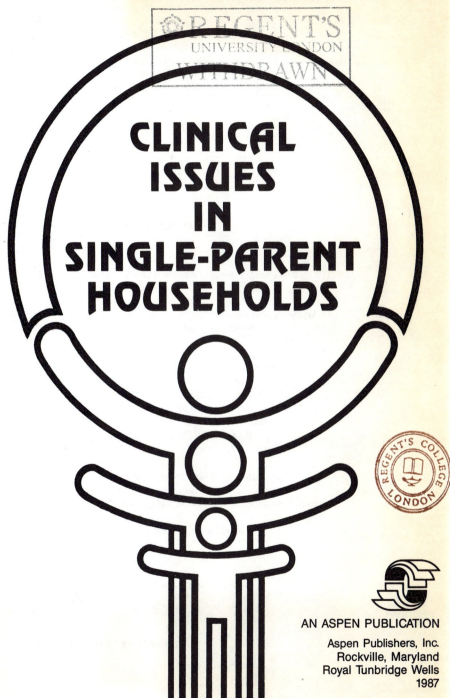

CLINICAL ISSUES IN SINGLE-PARENT HOUSEHOLDS

AN ASPEN PUBLICATION

Aspen Publishers, Inc.
Rockville, Maryland
Royal Tunbridge Wells
1987

Library of Congress Cataloging-in-Publication Data

Clinical issues in single-parent households.

(The Family therapy collections, ISSN: 0735-9152 ; 23)
"An Aspen publication."
Includes bibliographies and index.
1. Single parents—United States—Psychology.
2. Single-parent family—United States. 3. Family
psychotherapy—United States. I. Lindblad-Goldberg,
Marion. II. Series. [DNLM: 1. Family. 2. Family Therapy.
3. Parents. 4. Single Person. W1 FA454N v. 23 /
WM 430.5.F2 C6416]
HQ759.915.C59   1987   306.8′56   87-17502
ISBN: 0-89443-623-6

The Family Therapy Collections series is indexed in *Psychological
Abstracts* and the PsycINFO database

Article reprints are available from University Microfilms International,
300 North Zeeb Road, Dept., A.R.S., Ann Arbor, MI 48106.

Editorial Services: Ruth Bloom

Library of Congress Catalog Card Number: 87-17502
ISBN: 0-89443-623-6
ISSN: 0735-9152

Printed in the United States of America

1   2   3   4   5

Table of Contents

Board of Editors

Series Preface

Family Therapy Collection is a quarterly publication in which topics of current and specific interest to family therapists are presented. Each volume serves as a source of information for practicing therapists by translating theoretical and research conceptualizations into practical applications. Authored by practicing professionals, the articles in each volume provide in-depth coverage of a single aspect of family therapy.

This volume concentrates on single-parent households. Demographic data report increasing numbers of family households headed by one parent. The majority of single-parent homes are maintained by women. Single parents depend on a social support system involving family members and extrafamilial resources. It is an alternative family structure that meets the daily tasks of the members and encounters problems similar to nuclear families and some problems unique to a family with only one parent.

Family therapists are seeing an increasing number of families living with only one parent. A therapist profits from a conceptual framework to guide in the assessment and treatment planning with the family. Awareness of the impact of public policy on a single-parent household as well as the issues encountered by a single parent resolving a specific problem will assist a therapist in developing a perspective on each family. The articles in this volume have been designed to aid in developing such an awareness. The authors provide information about public policy, specific family experiences, and examples of practical methods in working with families.

Marion Lindblad-Goldberg, PhD is the editor of the volume. She has been an Associate Professor of Clinical Psychiatry and Director of the Family Therapy Center in the Department of Psychiatry at the University of Cincinnati. She is presently the Director of Family Therapy Training Center of the Philadelphia Child Guidance Clinic and an Associate Professor of Psychology in the Department of Psychiatry at the University of Pennsylvania. Dr.

Lindblad-Goldberg has specialized in research on single-parent families and received an ODHS Grant for a three year study of well-functioning and symptomatic low-income black single-parent families. This study has been significant in its focus on well-functioning single-parent households. In developing this volume, Dr. Lindblad-Goldberg has selected an outstanding group of authors who have presented stimulating concepts and illustrations that have practical implications for practicing family therapists.

James C. Hansen
Series Editor

Preface

The growth in the number of single-parent families during the last two decades has been dramatic, making the single-parent family a significant family form in today's society. Because the American family ideal for so long has been the two-parent household, insufficient knowledge about the single-parent family has created an abundance of myths and negative stereotypes. For example, use of the phrase "single-parent family" still conjures up the image of a "disintegrated" and therefore vulnerable unit despite evidence that many of the social/psychological problems associated with growing up in single-parent homes seem to be more a function of their poverty than of family structure per se. Additionally, the phrase "single-parent family" may inhibit professionals from exploring the role of the absent parent or other significant adult parental figures in the family system. To facilitate readability of the chapters in this volume, the phrase "single-parent family" is used; however, the volume is titled, *Clinical Issues of Single-Parent Households* to underscore the importance of accurately representing the membership of the household rather than defining the family system.

In selecting areas for inclusion in the volume an attempt was made to encompass the wide scope of this topic. In keeping with the high statistical frequency of low income female-headed families, the volume concentrates primarily on these families; however, a chapter on male-headed families is included in recognition of this developing family form. Not only is the variability in the precipitating event that created the single parenthood status (separation, divorce, death, and out-of-wedlock pregnancy) considered, but emphasis is placed on the diverse cultural backgrounds of these families.

The volume begins with a chapter by research demographers, McLanahan and Garfinkel, from the University of Wisconsin, and research clinician, Ooms, from Catholic University. These authors highlight the economic plight of female-headed families and the impact public policy has had in shaping the experiences of these families. This thought-provoking chapter explores possible causes for the increased single parent population and their poverty status. The current proposals of policymakers to connect child support, welfare reform, and employment and training programs are clearly elucidated so that clinicians can better appreciate the impact of these programs on mother-headed families.

Fulmer draws from his extensive clinical background at the Fordham-Tremont Community Mental Health Center in the South Bronx and at Albert Einstein College of Medicine. Working with low income, urban Puerto Rican and Black families, he presents an indepth discussion of the special problems of mourning within this population. He points out how poverty and the life cycle pattern of extended kinship family systems exposes families to unique types of losses. Fulmer's approach for assessing and treating unresolved mourning encompasses the extended family system. He uses this context to suggest appropriate focus and interventions during the stages of therapy.

A method for assessing the social networks and kinship systems of low-income, Black single-parent families is presented by Lindblad-Goldberg based on findings from a cross-sectional research study conducted at the Philadelphia Child Guidance Clinic. The importance of describing "healthy" functioning within this population is emphasized.

Expanding upon her impressive longitudinal research and clinical work at the Philadelphia Child Guidance Clinic in the area of difficult divorce processes, Isaacs illustrates the typical relationship patterns in which children find themselves after parental separation. As the children speak directly of their predicament in these dysfunctional situations, the clinician is alerted to the importance of helping divorcing families develop family patterns that best serve the child.

Two chapters are devoted to understanding the teenage single-parent family. Based on their innovative longitudinal study of low income, urban adolescent mothers conducted at the Philadelphia Child Guidance Clinic, Jemail and Nathanson discuss the relationship between family structural characteristics and adolescent adjustment to pregnancy. A lucid description of the stages families with a pregnant teen encounter is followed by a practical assessment and treatment plan clinicians can use to implement interventions designed to promote healthy adjustment. Gutierrez's sensitive and insightful descriptions of low income, Mainland Puerto Rican, teenage single parents is extracted from his research and clinical experiences with this cultural group at ASPIRA in Philadelphia, Pennsylvania. After providing the reader with a sociocultural rationale for the high rates of teenage pregnancy, he gives poignant case examples which detail the natural stages of the family's reactions to the pregnancy and the therapeutic interventions required at each stage.

Drawing both from his research and clinical experience at the Philadelphia Child Guidance Clinic, Jones offers a multifaceted examination of low income, never married, single mothers stressed by a young handicapped child. Clinical issues are identified and illustrated through diverse case material using an ecosystemic theoretical framework, encompassing the individual child, the family and personal network, and the professional network.

The "unchartered territory" of father-custody families is addressed in the closing chapter by Warshak of the University of Texas Health Science Center in Dallas. Combining both research and clinical knowledge, he offers a thorough articulation of family characteristics and factors mediating adjustment in these families. He further orients therapists to a variety of treatment goals and interventions which are effectively illustrated through case examples.

In conclusion, knowledge gleaned from this volume is intended to dispel current myths about single-parent households and replace them with an appreciation of the diversity and viability of the single-parent family unit.

Marion Lindblad-Goldberg
Volume Editor
August 1987

Acknowledgments

The authors have drawn on their distinguished professional experiences and I would like to thank them for their thoughtful and unique contributions to this volume. My deepest gratitude to Annalee who taught me about the strengths of single parent mothers.

Marion Lindblad-Goldberg

1. Female-Headed Families and Economic Policy: Expanding the Clinician's Focus

Sara S. McLanahan, PhD
Professor of Sociology
University of Wisconsin

Irwin Garfinkel, PhD
Professor of Social Work
University of Wisconsin

Theodora Ooms, MSW
Director, Family Impact Seminar
Catholic University of America
Washington, DC

F or the last two decades, those in the media have proclaimed that the American family is in crisis. There are many aspects to this perceived crisis, but clearly at its core is public concern about the rapid growth of families headed by single mothers. Although there is striking agreement among policy makers, analysts, and scholars on the nature of "the problem," there is considerable disagreement on possible solutions.

Part of the concern evolves from questions about the effects on children of divorce and the absence of fathers. Many doubt that one parent can do as good a job as can two parents. Most of the concern, however, is due to the realization that female-headed families are much more likely to be poor and dependent on public assistance than are two-parent families. Feminists have drawn attention to this so-called feminization of poverty, and child advocates have deplored the reemergence of staggering numbers of children in poverty after decades of antipoverty programs. In 1983, one of two children living in female-headed households was poor. In minority female-headed households, seven of ten children were poor (Congressional Budget Office, 1985).

The concern of policy makers is based not only on compassion for the welfare of poor mothers and their children, but also on the interests of the taxpayer: the increasing number of single-parent families is straining federal and state health and welfare budgets. One study estimated that teen-aged childbearing costs federal and state taxpayers $17 billion in health and welfare services each year (Burt, 1986).

1

THE SINGLE-PARENT POPULATION

Trends in the proportion of families headed by single women are quite similar for blacks and whites, although single motherhood has always been more common among blacks (Figure 1). Demographers estimate that approximately 45% of the white children and approximately 84% of the black children born in the late 1970s will live for some time with a single mother before they reach the age of 18. The median duration of residence in a female-headed household is 6 years for children of formerly married mothers and even longer for children born to never-married mothers. (Bumpass, 1984; Hofferth, 1985).

Historically, widowhood was the most common form of single parenthood. Since World War II, however, divorce and premarital birth have become increasingly important factors (Figure 2).

The distinction among these various types of single-parent families is important because these families differ considerably with respect to their access to

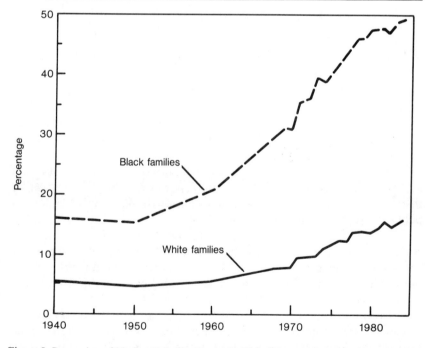

Figure 1 Proportion of Mother-Only Families in the United States, 1940–1984. *Source:* From *Single Mothers and Their Children* (p. 14) by I. Garfinkel and S. McLanahan, 1986, Washington, DC: The Urban Institute Press. Copyright 1986 by the Urban Institute. Reprinted with permission.

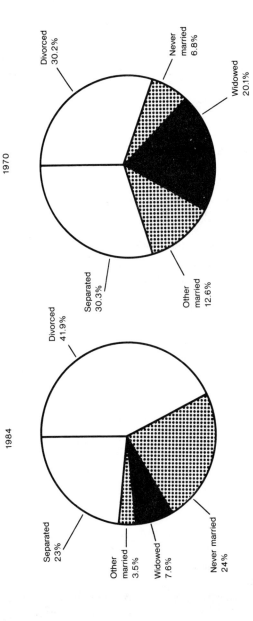

Note: The "other married" category refers to persons who report being married—as opposed to separated—but do not live with their spouse.

Figure 2 Children Living with One Parent, by Marital Status of Parent, 1970 and 1984. *Source*: U.S. Bureau of the Census, 1985.

economic and social resources. Widows have much higher incomes and experience less social disapproval than do other groups, whereas never-married mothers have the fewest resources of all single mothers and are most likely to become dependent on government welfare assistance.

Numerous explanations have been put forward to account for the growing number of female-headed families, and there are a great many empirical studies in which attempts have been made to test many of these arguments.

Increases in Welfare Benefits

In theory, higher welfare benefits increase the ability of single mothers to establish their own households. They enable a single mother to choose to keep her baby rather than to have an abortion or to surrender the baby for adoption. They also make it possible for poor married mothers to seek a divorce rather than to remain in a bad relationship. In short, all else being equal, increases in benefits should increase single motherhood. The size of the probable increase is not obvious, however.

Many studies have examined the relationship between welfare benefits and single motherhood to test this explanation for the increase in the number of these families. All together, these studies indicate that higher benefit levels do have some effect on living arrangements (e.g., encouraging subfamilies, such as a teen-aged mother and baby, to establish a separate household and discouraging remarriage). Higher benefits have much less effect on out-of-wedlock birth rates or divorce rates, however. Thus, the increase in welfare benefits between 1960 and 1975 can account for only an estimated 9% to 14% of the growth of female-headed families during this period (Garfinkel & McLanahan, 1986).

Increases in Women's Employment

Many people believe that the increase in single parenthood results from the entrance of so many married women with children into the labor force since World War II. Some people believe that the wider range of employment opportunities for women has created an "independence effect." Others, focusing on divorce alone, emphasize the "role conflict" that accompanies the renegotiation of traditional husband/wife roles when a wife becomes employed. Clearly, employment reduces a woman's economic dependence on her husband, as well as the amount of time that she has available to spend on housework and child care.

The empirical research in this area is nearly as voluminous as the literature on welfare. Preston and Richards (1975), for example, found that job opportunities, women's earnings, and men's unemployment rates are all good predictors of the marital status of women in the population. When jobs are available and women's wages are high relative to men's, women are less likely to be married. Several studies have indicated that married women who work or whose earnings potential is high are more likely to divorce than more dependent women are. Ross and Sawhill (1975), for example, calculated that a $1,000 increase in the earnings of married women is associated with a 7% increase in separation rates. Similarly, Cherlin (1976) found that the ratio of a wife's earnings capacity to her husband's earnings was a strong predictor of marital disruption. Taken together, these studies suggest that increased economic opportunities for women may account for a substantial part of the increase in single motherhood among whites. For black mothers, who have traditionally been employed in larger numbers than have white mothers, the overall effect of changes in women's employment opportunity is much smaller.

Decreases in Men's Employment

Changes in marital relationships as a result of unemployment were first documented in research on the Great Depression (Bakke, 1942; Komarovsky, 1940). More recently, Liebow (1967) vividly described how unemployment or underemployment undermined marital relationships and attitudes toward marriage among black men. Quantitative research has reinforced these findings in several areas. For example, researchers have shown that unemployment lowers psychological well-being, increases marital conflict, and sometimes even leads to family violence (Catalano & Dooley, 1977; Straus, Gelles, & Steinmetz, 1981).

Wilson and Neckerman (1986) developed an "index of marriageable males"—the ratio of black employed males per 100 black females of similar age in the population—that took into account not only unemployment, but also nonparticipation in the labor force and sex differences in mortality and incarceration rates. All these factors decrease the size of the "marriageable pool" of black men. Pointing to the decline in the number of unskilled jobs in cities such as New York, Philadelphia, and Baltimore, Wilson and Neckerman noted that such regions also showed the greatest increase in the number of female-headed families. They concluded that there is a correlation between these two trends. Based on their review of the evidence, Garfinkel and McLanahan (1986) hypothesized that the principal culprit in the decline in marriage among young blacks is the decline in male employment opportunities.

POVERTY OF FEMALE-HEADED FAMILIES AND ITS CAUSES

Roughly one of two single mothers is poor, according to the official government definition of poverty. Most of those who are not poor are economically insecure; many barely escape poverty. Nearly all divorced single mothers have experienced large drops in income. Duncan and Hoffman (1985) found that, one year after their divorce, the average income of the more fortunate half of divorced single mothers is equal to only 60% of their predivorce income.

Figure 3 shows trends in the prevalence of poverty for mother-only families, disabled persons, aged persons, and two-parent families for the years 1967 through 1983. These calculations took into account the assistance provided by the major government income support programs, such as Aid to Families with Dependent Children (AFDC), Social Security, and Disability Insurance. They did not include, however, the value of in-kind benefits, such as food stamps and Medicaid. Of all these groups, mother-only families have the highest percentage of poor families. The gap between mother-only families and other families has been widening because the economic position of the other groups has been improving.

A comparison of the sources of income available to different family types suggests three reasons that mother-only families are especially likely to be

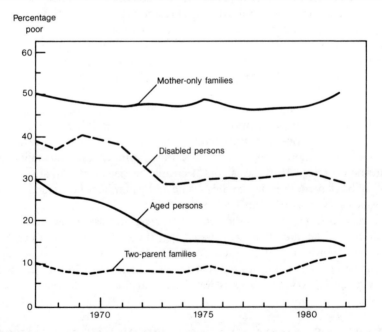

Figure 3 Poverty Rates for Mother-Only Families, the Aged, the Disabled, and Two-Parent Families, 1967–1982. *Source:* From *Single Mothers and Their Children* (p. 48) by I. Garfinkel and S. McLanahan, 1986, Washington, DC: The Urban Institute Press. Copyright 1986 by the Urban Institute. Reprinted with permission.

poor: (1) lower earnings of the family head, (2) lack of child support from the father, and (3) meager public assistance.

Low Earnings of Single Mothers

Accounting for approximately 60% to 70% of total income, the earnings of the household head are the major source of income for all family types, apart from those headed by widows. The ability of single mothers to earn income, therefore, is a critical determinant of their economic status. Female breadwinners earn only an estimated one-third as much as do married fathers, however, partly because they work fewer hours and partly because they have a lower hourly wage.

Only about 6% of single mothers who worked full-time year-round during the past decade were poor in any given year, as compared with more than 70% of nonworking women (Ellwood, 1985). To some extent, the apparent advantage of working mothers reflects the selection process that channels women with a higher earnings capacity into the labor force and women with a lower earnings capacity into homemaker and welfare status. On this point, Sawhill (1976) found that most of the women on welfare in the early 1970s had a very low earnings capacity and that, even if they worked full-time, more than 50% would still earn less than their welfare grants. There is good reason, therefore, to believe that a large proportion of women on welfare would be unable to earn their way out of poverty or significantly improve their economic position, even if they worked full-time all year.

The wage gap between women and men has not narrowed, and occupational segregation is still widespread. The median earnings of full-time, year-round women workers as a percentage of men's fell from 63.6% in 1955 to 60.2% in 1981 (Blau, 1984). The lower wage scale of women, then, is probably as important as their lower labor force participation rates in explaining the high incidence of poverty in mother-only families.

Inadequate Private Child Support

When a family splits, it loses the economies of scale that result from living together in one household. Even if the noncustodial father pays a reasonable amount of child support, the payments do not compensate fully for the costs that the separation entails. This is a moot point, however, as most noncustodial fathers do not pay reasonable amounts of child support.

National data on child support awards indicate that, in 1983, only about 58% of single mothers with children under 21 years old were awarded child support. Of these, only 50% received full payment, 26% received partial payment, and 24% received no payment at all (U.S. Bureau of the Census,

1986). Even when noncustodial fathers do pay child support, the amount paid is much lower than the contribution of either parent in two-parent families.

Inadequate Public Child Support

The United States is the only industrialized nation in the world that does not provide public cash allowances for all children. It also provides much less health care and day care than do most other industrialized nations. In fact, the United States is virtually unique in relying so heavily on welfare to aid female-headed families. The results of this policy are reflected in the contrast between the poverty status of widows and that of other single mothers. Fifty-one percent of all female-headed families (including widows) are poor, compared to 34% of families headed by widows. This difference is largely due to the difference in the benefits provided by Survivors Insurance, for which only widows are eligible, and those provided by AFDC, for which all single mothers are eligible. The average level of benefits in Survivors Insurance is much higher than the average level of welfare benefits. Furthermore, the proportion of widows who receive Survivors Insurance is much higher than the proportion of other single mothers who receive welfare. Finally, benefits for a widowed mother are reduced by only 50% of earnings if she works, and benefits for the child are not reduced at all if she either works or remarries.

There are many serious problems with the AFDC program that contribute to its failure to lift single mothers out of poverty. Benefit levels and eligibility criteria are set by the states and, thus, vary widely. Because AFDC benefits are not indexed to inflation, their value falls in real terms every year if states fail to enact increases in benefits. Moreover, the fact that eligibility for AFDC benefits also entitles single-parent families to Medicaid constitutes a serious disincentive to becoming independent of welfare, because the kinds of jobs available to AFDC recipients do not usually carry health insurance. Finally, by drastically reducing benefits as earnings increase, welfare programs replace rather than supplement earnings. The choice faced by poor single mothers is not an attractive one: (1) become dependent on welfare or (2) work full-time to achieve, at best, a marginally better economic position and risk losing valuable in-kind benefits such as Medicaid and public housing.

RECENT CHANGES IN POLICIES

Many of the psychosocial problems of children who grow up in families headed by single women are due to the economic insecurity and poverty in which they live. The government can reduce these problems by increasing the incomes of poor families in general and mother-only families in particular.

Several features of the Income Tax Reform Act of 1986 were aimed at reducing the tax liabilities of poor families and, thus, increasing their income. Of these, the two most important were increasing the personal exemption from $1,080 to $2,000 and liberalizing the earned income tax credit. The government may also alleviate poverty by increasing benefits in the various income support programs, such as the AFDC program, and improving the collection of private child support payments.

Policy makers are faced with a difficult dilemma, as increasing program benefits may lead to an increase in the number of AFDC-eligible families and the length of time that these families depend on government assistance. In order to avoid this undesirable result, most current experiments or proposals for alleviating the poverty of female-headed families encourage or require single mothers to work.

Reduction in Welfare Benefits

Between 1955 and 1975, the real value of welfare benefits for female-headed families doubled. Between 1975 and 1980, however, inflation cut the value of all benefits received by mother-only families by approximately 13%. The Reagan Administration in 1981 decided to try to reduce welfare dependence (rather than poverty per se) by decreasing benefits and tightening eligibility. Congress eventually adopted benefit cuts, that were more modest than those originally proposed by the Administration, but reduced benefits to mother-only families by another 12% (Garfinkel & McLanahan, 1986). Taken together, the reductions in benefits to families headed by single women between 1975 and 1985 have been substantial, eradicating more than one-fourth of the increases that had been obtained during the previous two decades. Welfare recipients who worked were hurt especially hard by these cuts (Garfinkel & McLanahan, 1986).

Work Requirements for Mothers

Until the early 20th century, single mothers were expected to work. For the next half-century, the stated objective of government income support programs was to provide single mothers with enough aid to enable them to stay home and look after their children, as middle-class mothers did. Not until the late 1960s, however, was that objective achievable. By that time, married middle-class mothers were entering the labor force in large numbers, and poor single mothers were increasingly expected to work as well.

At first, the federal government tried to induce AFDC mothers to work by creating work incentives within AFDC. The Reagan Administration rejected this approach in favor of a pure work requirement, seeking to cut off benefits to those who worked—thus forcing them to manage on their own resources—and to require those who received benefits to work for them. By the mid-1980s, Congress had agreed to much, but not all, of this strategy. Currently, almost every major welfare reform proposal contains both work requirements and provisions for services, such as training and day care, that make it possible for welfare recipients to work.

In order to enforce work requirements, the government must create or locate jobs. Some have argued that it is not feasible to enforce work requirements when the unemployment rate is higher than 7% (U.S. General Accounting Office, 1985), but a number of states have already demonstrated their ability to create and find jobs. Apart from the issue of technical feasibility, it is necessary to determine whether the benefits of enforcing work requirements offset the costs. Studies generally indicate that, although work and training programs for women who head families do cost more initially in comparison to the payment of cash benefits only, gains in earnings are sufficiently large to make the programs profitable within 3 to 4 years (Bassi & Ashenfelter, 1986; Hollister, Kemper, & Maynard, 1984). Initial costs are higher than welfare costs because both the cost of finding or creating jobs and the cash benefit must be paid.

The actual increase in the incomes of single mothers is smaller than the increase in earnings that may result from the enforcement of a work requirement, because they lose some benefits and have a number of work-related expenses, such as child care and transportation. Whether AFDC families realize gains or losses from the enforcement of work requirements depends on the nature of the key programs that aid poor single mothers and the attractiveness and availability of jobs in the regular labor market. Given the choice, many mothers may choose the combination of lower income from welfare and more time for child-rearing, housework, and leisure.

There are three reasons for caution in interpreting the evidence in favor of compulsory work programs. First, programs that involve significant elements of compulsion may be less profitable both to the beneficiaries and to society as a whole because unwilling workers are likely to be less productive and more costly to supervisors. Second, and even more important, the child care costs for preschool children may easily be so high as to offset the short-term earnings gains of the program. Third, it may be unrealistic to expect single mothers to work full-time year-round—as they must in order to be self-supporting—when such complete labor force participation is the exception rather than the rule among married mothers. Given the fact that work requirements impose a dual role on a single mother (i.e., care-giver and breadwinner), requiring single mothers to work for their welfare checks is to place a heavy burden on them. In doing so, the country should proceed cautiously, with concern for the well-being of both the children and their mothers.

To a clinician, one of the most encouraging features of the welfare reform debate is that many of the current proposals recognize the realities of the lives of welfare families. Whereas once the AFDC clients were referred to as "able-bodied recipients," they are now more often called "single mothers." Proposals couple work requirements with the provision of necessary services, such as child care, training, and transportation. The American Public Welfare Administration (APWA) has recommended the institution of a services contract that specifies the mutual, feasible responsibilities of the AFDC program and the welfare recipient. Indeed, some of the proposals suggest that single mothers should be required to work only part-time or enter some limited training program.

Child Support

In 1984, Congress unanimously enacted legislation that requires all states (1) to enact laws that withhold from wages all future child support payments once the obligor is delinquent in payments for 1 month and (2) to appoint commissions to design statewide guidelines for child support standards. The original impetus for such child support legislation arose from the desire of policy makers to recoup some of the expenses of the AFDC program. All AFDC mothers are now required to cooperate in identifying and locating the absent fathers of their children, unless doing so is proved to be detrimental to their welfare or to the welfare of their children. The states use collections from these efforts to defray AFDC expenditures. Indeed, states have begun to recover 2 to 3 dollars for every dollar spent on administering the program.

Although earlier federal child support laws had permitted the use of these collection services by nonwelfare families, there were no fiscal incentives to encourage state governments to expend any effort on collections for non-welfare families. The 1984 legislation was enacted partly in response to pressure from advocacy organizations that were becoming aware of the serious problems of nonpayment of child support in nonwelfare families and of the sharp drop in income of divorced custodial mothers. The new legislation provided incentives to ensure that states made their various services (e.g., paternity testing and establishment, the computerized federal parent locator service), and the collection mechanisms available to both welfare and non-welfare families. Although states may charge nonwelfare families a modest fee for the services, the child support enforcement system is now available to all custodial parents.

If all potentially eligible children obtained a child support award based on some agreed upon standard, and if all such children received the full amount due them, the incomes of families headed by women would increase by more than $10 billion. Welfare caseloads would decrease by 25%. Even 100%

collection of all child support obligations derived from any reasonable standard would leave the overwhelming majority of AFDC recipients no better off than they were without the program, however, because most noncustodial parents of AFDC children do not earn enough to pay as much child support as their children are already receiving in AFDC benefits.

Uses of Increased Child Support Collections. Most of the increases in child support collections for families on welfare accrue to the government in the form of AFDC savings. At this time, there are two methods of sharing a portion of the collected funds with AFDC families. Congress has required all states to ignore the first $50 per month of the child support payment in calculating AFDC grants. This requirement modestly increases the incomes of mother-only families on AFDC in which there is a noncustodial father who makes child support payments. It also slightly increases the number of mother-only families that continue to receive AFDC.

Alternatively, the increased child support collections may be used to help fund a nonwelfare benefit that encourages work. This approach is being pursued on a demonstration basis in the state of Wisconsin. Under the Wisconsin child support assurance system, child support obligations are set as a fixed percentage of the noncustodial parent's gross income: 17% for one child, 25% for two, 29% for three, 31% for four, and 34% for five or more children. The obligation is withheld from wages and other sources of income in all cases, just as income and payroll taxes are withheld. The child receives the money paid by the noncustodial parent or an assured child support benefit, whichever is greater. Thus, the savings in AFDC that result from increased child support collections are funneled back into the system in the form of an assured benefit to increase the economic well-being of families with children eligible for child support. According to Garfinkel and McLanahan (1986), such a program could reduce proverty among American families potentially eligible for child support by 40% and AFDC caseloads by more than 50% at no extra cost to the taxpayer.

One criticism of the Wisconsin child support assurance program is that it will benefit only those AFDC mothers who work. In most states for those who are unable to work, who cannot find jobs, or who simply prefer to take care of their children full-time, the program provides less than AFDC. Thus, the success of the child support assurance approach hinges largely on the availability of jobs and the extent to which poor custodial mothers (as well as poor noncustodial fathers) work.

Whatever the merits of particular proposals, there is clearly a growing interest among policy makers in connecting child support, welfare reform, and employment and training programs. This multipronged approach is complex and may be very difficult to implement. It emphasizes a partnership model in which both parents—noncustodial and custodial—are expected to be responsible for child support. Their efforts are to be encouraged and supplemented, not supplanted by government support and services.

Unwed Fathers. While the federal child support program requirements apply equally to the once-married and the never-married, unwed fathers are seldom involved by the system. Unlike the once-married fathers, whose paternity is not in question, unwed fathers are liable for support only after paternity has been established. State and local studies suggest that, while many unwed fathers may informally admit to paternity and contribute small amounts of support, paternity is formally established and child support awarded in fewer than two of ten cases. (Blood tests to establish paternity are now 97% reliable.)

Most social service and health care personnel who work with young unwed mothers know very little about the child support program. Moreover, they perceive the child support system as punitive and are unlikely to encourage the unwed mother to establish paternity. These personnel rarely contact the unwed father; should they do so, they do not focus on issues of child support or paternity.

Among the major barriers to establishing paternity are the attitudes of the unwed mothers and their families, who quite often want nothing to do with the father, make no efforts to establish paternity, and do not cooperate effectively in attempts to locate the father. It is generally agreed, however, that young fathers should be encouraged to make payments of at least token or in-kind support and that they should be offered the opportunity, or even required, to enroll in training and employment programs so that they will eventually be able to fulfill their financial responsibilities (Smollar & Ooms, 1987).

A project to study the impact of the child support system and other policies on young unwed fathers revealed a number of reasons that child support was seldom collected from unwed fathers (Smollar & Ooms, 1987). It was clear, for example, that state officials gave these cases very low priority, in part because the collection of child support from these fathers was very time-consuming and produced only small amounts of financial support in the short run. (Many were still in school or had dropped out of school and were unemployed.) This de facto policy of neglect is coming under growing criticism as the financial benefits that may accrue to the child and mother in the long run (e.g., when the father becomes employed or joins the military service) and the child's right to know his father are being recognized.

One further dilemma that pervades the issue of child support is the extent to which support payments are seen to be tied to visitation. Research on this issue is scarce, and the findings are somewhat contradictory. Opinions are strong, however. Although they have little evidence, men's rights groups declare that men do not pay child support because they are denied access to their children. On the other hand, anecdotal evidence suggests that custodial mothers are sometimes reluctant to establish paternity or to push for child support lest the father claim visitation rights that they are not prepared to cede.

IMPLICATIONS FOR CLINICIANS

The relationship of single-parent families, especially those headed by women, to other social systems is profoundly shaped by their precarious economic situation. This financial stress affects not only the single mother's pattern of work, but also her contacts with welfare and child support agencies, school personnel, and health care providers. Financial matters are frequently the source of tension and conflict among the mother, the child(ren)'s father, and the extended families. It is very important that clinicians who observe these difficulties in single-parent families understand that these difficulties are widely shared by single parents and are not the products of a particular family's dysfunction. Furthermore, when clinicians work to empower single-parent families and help them mobilize sources of support, they need to be aware of the complex facts and issues involved and the programs available.

Clinicians who work with families in which a young woman has a baby out of wedlock should be aware that there is a growing trend to enforce the financial responsibilities and assure the rights of unwed fathers. Already, unwed fathers have clearly recognized rights to veto a mother's plans to have the baby adopted. It has been proposed that paternity be established at birth for all out-of-wedlock children, which may involve putative fathers at an earlier stage in decision making about the child. This trend is likely to be resisted by those who believe that the unwed mother should be able to choose whether to name the father and claim support from him. However, family-oriented clinicians should understand the need to balance the claims of the child, the mother, the father, and the family.

It is common for single mothers to receive welfare for at least a short period of time, but it too often becomes a sustained way of life. Although welfare provides some measure of economic stability and health care, many believe that the experience is stigmatizing and detrimental to the family's self-image. In addition, the frequent changes in eligibility criteria and benefits, as well as the inherent complexity of the system, create a bureaucratic jungle of rules and regulations that imposes enormous burdens on welfare mothers and welfare workers alike. Clinicians should be aware that, in the future, there will be increasing pressure on welfare mothers to enter training programs or obtain employment. This will create additional pressures on these mothers to find alternative sources of child care and will add more stress—though perhaps also more satisfaction—to their lives.

The double duty of single mothers exacerbates the problems that all employed parents face in balancing the responsibilities of work and family. While society no longer frowns on single mothers for working (Schorr & Moen, 1979), many social institutions important to mothers, such as schools and medical clinics, operate on schedules that make no allowance for mothers who work. In single-parent households, accommodations to these schedules are not usually possible unless members of the extended family are available to act as surrogate parents. Too often, the working mother's lack of flexibility (and income) means that she does not take her child to the doctor until sickness turns into an emergency. Too often, her failure to become involved in school activities, to keep school appointments, or to participate in conferences is interpreted by school personnel as a lack of interest in her child's progress (Morawetz & Walker, 1984).

Happily, some school staffs are showing a much greater awareness of the special needs of single-parent families. They are becoming much more flexible in their expectations and are modifying their curricula. Increasingly, policies permit and even encourage school personnel routinely to share information about the child's progress and the school program with the noncustodial parent (Henderson, Marburger, & Ooms, 1985).

Some employers—but still only a fraction—are also becoming more responsive to the special needs of employed single parents (Axel, 1985). Cafeteria style fringe benefits offer subsidies for child care, more generous maternity leave, and family leave. More employers, both public and private, offer part-time work without loss of benefits and seniority.

The consideration of single-parent families as a problem for social policy is not a symptom of zealous moralism, but a realistic and constructive position. Most policy makers readily admit that many single mothers surmount their economic and other difficulties to become good parents. Focusing attention on the economic problems of single-parent families in the aggregate is a necessary and welcomed step towards developing sound policies and programs to help single mothers.

REFERENCES

Axel, H. (1985). *Corporations and families: Changing practices and perspectives* (Report No. 868). New York: The Conference Board.

Bakke, E.W. (1942). *Citizens without work*. New Haven: Yale University Press.

Bassi, L.J., & Ashenfelter, O. (1986). The effect of direct job creation and training programs on low-skilled workers. In S.H. Danziger & D.H. Weinberg (Eds.), *Fighting poverty: What works and what doesn't* (pp. 133–151). Cambridge, MA: Harvard University Press.

Blau, F.D. (1984). Occupational segregation and labor market discrimination. In B.F. Reskin (Ed.), *Sex segregation in the workplace: Trends, explorations, remedies* (pp. 117–143). Washington, DC: National Academy Press.

Bumpass, L.L. (1984). Children and marital disruption: A replication and update. *Demography*, *21*, 71–82.

Burt, M. (1986). *Estimates of public costs for teenage childbearing*. Unpublished paper prepared for the Center for Population Options, Washington, DC.

Catalano, R., & Dooley, C.D. (1977). Economic predictions of depressed mood and stressful life events in a metropolitan community. *Journal of Health and Social Behavior, 18*, 292–307.

Cherlin, A. (1976). *Social and economic determinants of marital separation*. Unpublished doctoral dissertation, University of California, Los Angeles.

Congressional Budget Office. (1985). *Reducing poverty among children*. Washington, DC: Congress of the United States.

Duncan, G.J., & Hoffman, S. (1985, October). *Welfare dynamics and welfare policy: Past evidence and future research directions*. Paper presented at the annual meeting of the Association for Public Policy Analysis and Management, Washington, DC.

Ellwood, D. (1985). *Targeting the would-be long-term recipients of AFDC: Who should be served?* Unpublished preliminary report, Harvard University.

Garfinkel, I., & McLanahan, S. (1986). *Single mothers and their children: A new American dilemma?* Washington, DC: The Urban Institute.

Henderson, A., Marburger, C., & Ooms, T. (1985). *Beyond the bake sale: An educator's guide to working with parents*. Columbia, Md, National Committee for Citizens in Education.

Hofferth, S. (1985). Updating children's life course. *Journal of Marriage and the Family, 47*, 93–116.

Hollister, R.G., Jr., Kemper, P., & Maynard, R. (1984). *The National Supported Work Demonstration*. Madison: The University of Wisconsin Press.

Komarovsky, M. (1940). *The unemployed man and his family*. New York: Octagon Books.

Liebow, E. (1967). *Talley's corner*. Boston: Little, Brown and Co.

Morawetz, A., & Walker, G. (1984). *Brief therapy with single parent families*. New York: Bruner/Mazel.

Preston, S.H., & Richards, A.T. (1975). The influence of women's work opportunities on marriage rates. *Demography, 12*, 209–222.

Ross, H., & Sawhill, I. (1975). *Time of transition: The growth of families headed by women*. Washington, DC: The Urban Institute.

Sawhill, I. (1976). Discrimination and poverty among women who head families. *Signs, 2*, 201–211.

Schorr, A., & Moen, P. (1979). The single parent and public policy. *Social Policy, 15*, 15–21.

Smollar, J., & Ooms, T. (1987). *Young unwed fatherhood: Research review, policy dilemmas and options*. Project report from the Office of the Assistant Secretary for Planning and Evaluation, U.S. Department of Health and Human Services, Washington, DC.

Straus, M.A., Gelles, R., & Steinmetz, S. (1981). *Behind closed doors*. New York: Anchor Books.

U.S. Bureau of the Census. (1985). *Marital status and living arrangements: March 1984* (Current Population Reports, Series P-20, No. 399). Washington, DC: U.S. Government Printing Office.

U.S. Bureau of the Census. (1986). *Child support and alimony: 1983* (Current Population Reports, Special Studies Series P-23, No. 148). Washington, DC: U.S. Government Printing Office.

U.S. General Accounting Office. (1985, August). *Evidence is insufficient to support the administration's proposed changes to AFDC work programs*. U.S. General Accounting Office Report to the

Chairman, Subcommittee on Intergovernmental Relations and Human Resources, House of Representatives Committee on Government Operations.

Wilson, W.J., & Neckerman, K.M. (1986). Poverty and family structure: the widening gap between evidence and public policy issues. In S.H. Danziger & D.H. Weinberg (Eds.), *Fighting poverty: What works and what doesn't* (pp. 232–259). Cambridge, MA: Harvard University Press.

2. Special Problems of Mourning in Low-Income Single-Parent Families

Richard H. Fulmer, PhD
Director, Family Therapy Training Program
Fordham-Tremont Community Mental Health Center
and Assistant Clinical Professor
Department of Psychiatry
Albert Einstein College of Medicine
Bronx, New York

The structure of the single-parent family and the process by which it becomes one create a context in which it is especially difficult to mourn (Fulmer, 1983). Thus, unresolved mourning may be a source of the depression frequently observed in single mothers, particularly those in the lower income groups. Children in these families may show symptoms in response to this depression, further overwhelming their mothers and contributing to their depressive discouragement.

The kinship network of low-income families and the way they pass through the family life cycle expose them to unique types of losses and protect them from others. The frequency and intensity of negative environmental pressures at once gives low-income families more occasions to mourn and depletes their capacity to do so. Because the practical, physical effects of loss are so critical in low-income families, the psychic effects of necessary compensatory measures may go unrecognized, and uncompleted mourning may become the norm.

The clinical observations that form the basis for this chapter were made in a community mental health center in the south Bronx, an impoverished area of one of the boroughs of New York City. The patient population served there is 55% Hispanic (predominantly Puerto Rican), 30% black and 14% white; 85% of these families receive public assistance.

The author wishes to express his gratitude to Ron Taffel, PhD, for his very helpful comments on earlier versions of this chapter.

Middle class families usually become single parent families by the following sequence: the couple marries, establishes a home separate from their parents, and has children. It is then that the two-generational nuclear unit loses the husband/father through death, desertion or divorce. Middle income mothers usually attempt to maintain the nuclear household without a husband.

Some low-income families become female-headed by that sequence, but may do so by a different process—conceiving out of wedlock during adolescence. Disadvantaged young women, regardless of race, are three to four times more likely to become unwed mothers than middle income adolescents (Children's Defense Fund, 1986).

LIFE CYCLE ACCELERATION IN THE LOW-INCOME FAMILY

Disadvantaged adolescent girls have little reason to expect fulfillment in school or work, so they have little incentive to delay pregnancy. Thus in a large percentage of low-income families, a girl's first pregnancy occurs quite early, preceding marriage and even preceding an extended courtship. Unless the girl's family makes a special effort to include him, the young father has no role in the new family. If the girl is young, the couple is unlikely to marry or even to live together. Therefore, the couple never establishes itself as a unit that is independent from parents or children.

Because the young, unemployed, undereducated mother cannot support herself and her child, and because she can rely even less on her boyfriend for support, she often continues to live with her family of origin. In a study of a predominantly Black group of 320 low-income single mothers in Baltimore, Furstenberg (1981) found that, during their first pregnancy, "90% lived with a parent or close relative. One year after delivery, 77% were still doing so. Even five years after the birth of their child, 46% remained with their parents or other kin. At that time, only 26% were married" (p. 137). When the couple relationship is not developed or highly invested, the loss of the husband/father is not a trauma of the same severity that it is for middle-income families and does not need to be mourned in the same way.

THE KINSHIP NETWORK: ISSUES OF RACE, CULTURE, AND SOCIAL CLASS

The term *single-parent families* is something of a misnomer for adolescent mothers and their children in low-income families. These girls do not raise their children alone. Remaining at home, these adolescent girls blend their infants into the subgroup of their own younger siblings. As head of the household, the adolescent's mother (now a grandmother) has primary authority in raising her daughter's children. This family is a "kinship network" (Stack, 1974) or "extended family" (Martin & Martin, 1978) in which three or more generations share child care responsibilities and help each other as needed and as possible according to the resources of the family. If one mother is in difficult circumstances, her sister or her aunt is expected to do more than just babysit. She may very well move some or all of the mother's children into her home and care for them until the mother can do so again herself. Teen-aged mothers in these kinship networks do not become single parents by the *loss* of the husband/father, because they were never established as part of a couple.

Winch and Blumberg (1971) contend that because this family form is so prevalent in contemporary society, the father-absent kinship network should not be considered an abnormal or "disorganized" example of "social pathology" (p. 139). Rather they suggest it be considered as one among a set of family types, each of which requires an explanation.

Most American sociological scholarship on this family form has been written about black families. Hispanic families have a different culture and history in the Americas and may exhibit some important differences. However, in recent years low income members of these two minorities have been sharing the same residential areas and environmental conditions in American cities and may also share important similarities in the function of the extended family. For instance, in both black (Stack, 1974) and Puerto Rican (Garcia-Preto, 1982) families, children are seen as the responsibility of the whole kinship network, not just the biological mother. Fosterage and informal adoption of kin are common in low-income families of both races. Rogler and his associates (1983, p. 22) write that Puerto Rican families in Puerto Rico "enmesh their members in a system of help-giving exchanges," a characteristic very similar to descriptions of black families.

A number of sociologists consider the prevalence of the kinship network to be a function of the degree to which a particular culture has been successful at getting jobs in industrialized society (Goode, 1963; Gutman, 1978). To the extent that low-income men and women achieve stable employment, they tend toward the nuclear family model with its delay of pregnancy and emphasis on the centrality of the couple. When they are subject to the environmental pressures of unemployment and racism, they use the kinship model to share scarce resources. Thus the kinship network is not itself a problem, but an attempt at a solution to a problem.

THE FAMILY LIFE CYCLE IN A KINSHIP NETWORK

Infancy

When it is working well, such an extended family structure may well be a very good one for infants. The inexperienced solitary mother of the middle income nuclear family may become overwhelmed by having to handle the learning and practice of childrearing in a relatively isolated condition (Minturn & Lambert, 1964). In a kinship network, however, the low-income infant may enjoy several experienced caretakers who can support and teach its own mother.

Toddlerhood

This relatively positive stage may end, however, when the children begin to toddle. They take up much more space in cramped apartments. More importantly, they learn to say "no" and require discipline. Caring for them is a more exhausting, less rewarding experience and the number of willing volunteers around the house may dwindle rapidly (Furstenberg, 1981). As issues of authority become primary for the child, conflict between grandmother and daughter may arise in parallel process around the issue of "who's in charge?" The grandmother may become critical of her daughter and the child may show symptoms that are a function of a "parental" division between mother and grandmother.

LOSSES ASSOCIATED WITH FAMILY STRUCTURE IN LATER LIFE CYCLE STAGES

Establishment of a Couple

As low-income teen-aged mothers mature, they may wish to set up their own households. They marry or begin living with a man for the first time, moving out and taking their children with them. While this is a developmental achievement for the mother, it may be a major loss for her children. Up to this point, they have been living in a household headed by their grandmother. She may have been their most reliable care-giver. A separation from or loss of grandmother is thus a more significant event for children of low-income families than it would be for middle-income children.

The mother's marriage, even if it is her first, creates a stepfamily. She loves her husband, but her children have no reason to be especially happy about the marriage. They are losing their grandmother and gaining an adult male stranger. If this stranger brings his own children into the family, the mother's children may also lose their customary sibling position. When their mother and stepfather begin having children of their own, the mother's children may lose additional status if their stepfather becomes more attached to his natural children. It is probably impossible to avoid such losses for the children. The biggest problems occur when these losses are not recognized. Mourning reactions, especially in children, must be acknowledged and supported by the family if they are to run their course and be resolved. There is a special risk in low-income single-parent families that the children's losses will go unnoticed and emerge in symptomatic behavior.

The young mother's decision to establish a separate household is also a loss for the grandmother. In some cases, the grandmother has simply refused to let the mother take her (the mother's) eldest child, saying "you didn't raise him, and you can't take him now." It is a measure of the grandmother's power in such families that she can do this without the censure (and perhaps with the tacit approval) of the kinship network.

This transition to a couple-based nuclear family is difficult for the whole kinship network. Because there are so few reliable employment opportunities for urban minority men, it is very difficult for nuclear family units to endure. Stack (1974) wrote that, because of this economically based instability, "the kinship network regard(s) any marriage as both a risk to the woman and her children and as a threat to the durability of the kin group" (p. 117).

Separation

Women who enter a marriage with a child conceived or born out of wedlock have significantly higher rates of marital disruption (O'Connell & Rogers, 1984). If separation occurs, the various children of the family may have very different mourning responses. Those originally raised by the mother and the grandmother may not be sad to see their stepfather go, whereas his natural children may be very unhappy. Recognizing and tolerating the variety of mourning responses in the sibling subgroups are special challenges for the mother, for other care-giving adults, and for the siblings themselves. This loss may be an even more poignant one for the mother, because she has lost a man with whom she had hoped to create an enduring household.

Changes in the Sibling Subsystems

Another potential source of loss due to family structure that is especially common in lower income single parent families is the changeability of the sibling subsystem. When mother cannot take care of her children because of her youth, financial reversals, having an infant, getting a job, losing an apartment, an episode of drug use, or being unable to control an adolescent, another member of the kinship network may informally "adopt" some or all of her children. In addition to the change of executive, the mother's establishment of a household also means a change in residence for the children, perhaps even a change in neighborhood or geographical region. In a study of Black adolescent girls, Gibbs (1986) found that depression was positively correlated with their families' geographical mobility.

In the middle-income group, even in single-parent families, it is expected that the siblings in low-income families rarely stay together throughout childhood. If the mother can handle some, but not all, of her children, the sibling group may be divided, some staying with their mother and some staying with other relatives in the kinship network. In some cases, the younger children have been virtually raised by an older sister, and separation from this sister may be a catastrophic loss for them. No one perceives such separations as ideal, but circumstances may necessitate them. As always, the danger is that adult family members may (understandably) hope and expect that, if the child is provided for and emergencies are handled, the child should be happy and satisfied. They may not recognize (or may recognize but be intolerant of) mourning reactions.

As she becomes older and more competent, the low-income single mother may begin to care for relatives' children, including her own daughter's. She may take in foster children as a means of supporting herself and her own children. These changes may enrich or impoverish individual siblings. Their effect, if any, can be discovered only through specific inquiry and observation.

VULNERABILITY TO DEPRESSION IN LOW-INCOME FAMILIES

The second way in which low-income single-parent families differ from middle-income single-parent families is that low-income families experience greater severity and frequency of traumatic life events, such as unemployment, disease, crime, accidents, and other environmental intrusions. Furthermore, they are seldom able to protect themselves against these traumas; they have no cash reserves, no insurance, few jobs, and few connections in the legal and medical worlds. The effect of the great number of traumas and the paucity of reparative resources accumulates, draining the psychic resources of these families and making low-income mothers (Belle et al., 1979) and their daughters (Gibbs, 1986) vulnerable to depression.

Brown and Harris (1978) studied a sample of women living in London and found that working-class women were four times more likely to be depressed than were middle-class women, even when the severity of the precipitating trauma (what Brown and Harris called the "provoking agent") was the same. According to Brown and Harris, four factors contribute to women's vulnerability to depression:

1. loss of their mother before the age of 11
2. lack of a job

3. lack of a confiding relationship with a husband or boyfriend
4. three or more children under age 14 at home

They showed that women become depressed at a much higher rate when these factors are present, regardless of the severity of their current loss. The effects they discovered should be even more extreme for those who have even fewer resources than those working-class mothers had. Brown and Harris hypothesized that the accumulation of past losses and current stress factors engender a feeling of hopelessness that makes the impact of current loss much greater. They concluded, therefore, that the crucial causative factor in depression is not grief itself, but the hopelessness that precedes grief.

Similarly, Deutsch (1937) stated that, if grief runs its normal course, no depression will result. The mourning process may be blocked, however, if the ego is already depleted by other painful experiences at the time of the loss. Those individuals already vulnerable because of such experiences may find mourning intolerably painful and, thus, defend themselves by appearing not to grieve at all. Deutsch believed that unresolved grief would be expressed indirectly in some manner (i.e., a symptom). Her model for this dynamic process within the individual can be applied to the family system. When one family member is experiencing a defensive "absence of grief," it may be expressed in the symptomatic actions of another family member.

LOSS-RELATED SYMPTOMS

Multiple and severe losses are almost inevitable for low-income families. Given their limited resources for recovery, these families should be considered at special risk for loss-related symptoms. A number of symptoms displayed by the children brought for treatment may be related to the family's response to its losses.

Loss of a Parent, Maternal Depression, and Delinquency

Bowlby (1967) reviews work that establishes a strong correlation between a child's early (between ages 0–9) loss of a parent through death, divorce, desertion or prolonged absence and repeated delinquency during adolescence. Weissman (1983) agrees that the absence of a parent with whom to identify may contribute to delinquency by interfering with the development of the child's conscience. She extends this idea to include the children of depressed mothers as well, suggesting that although mother is physically present, her withdrawal and detachment may be experienced by the adolescent as a loss not only of nurturance but of direction and control. Delinquency, especially gang involvement, may counteract consequent feelings of helplessness (p. 109).

Hoffman (1981) suggests another dynamic by which maternal depression may be related to apparent behavior disorders in children. She describes interviews of low-income families by Minuchin et al. (1967) and Aponte (then unpublished, now presented in Aponte [1986]) in which children seem to be acting in a chaotic and unruly manner. She contends that the children are practicing "collusive mischief" (pp. 82–84) by creating a disturbance in one case to get a temporarily absent mother to return to the room and in another case to rouse a depressed mother out of lethargy into watchful anger. She suggests that children who are made anxious by maternal silence and learn to activate mother in this way may tend to repeat this pattern in school whenever a teacher is sitting quietly (for example, marking papers). The children may perceive a teacher so engaged to be depressed, misbehave to rouse her, and thereby, become reputed as impulsive and delinquent.

Drug Abuse

Coleman, Kaplan, and Downing (1986) interviewed ex–heroin addicts, college students, and psychiatric patients and found a significantly higher incidence of death and separation in the backgrounds of heroin addicts and their parents. According to these researchers, few addicts' families have religious beliefs or a sense of higher purpose that can help them in mourning these losses. Because mourning is unresolved, any separation is likely to disrupt these families. When the children reach adolescence and the family is faced with the life cycle task of helping them leave home, heroin abuse "provides the family with a defense against hopelessness and despair" (p. 6). The addict comes into conflict with the parents and either leaves home or is expelled precipitously. Because of the heroin abuse, the addict functions poorly in the outside world, becomes debilitated, and returns home to recuperate when his or her resources are expended. Like Stanton and Todd (1982), Coleman and her associates saw this pattern repeated many times in the lives of addicts and concluded that these addicts are not solitary "street people," but "actually very connected to home and family, even if this tie is associated with inordinate anxiety" (Coleman et al., 1986, p. 20).

Coleman and her colleagues' research unfortunately does not control for the different socioeconomic status of their three comparison groups. Because the socioeconomic status of their addict group was almost surely lower than that of their college student group, it is difficult to determine whether the addiction was a consequence of unresolved mourning or of the general stresses of growing up under the conditions of poverty in a neighborhood where drugs were readily available. The clinical findings of Coleman (1980) and Stanton

(1977) are persuasive, however, and suggest that the clinician should at least search for a family pattern of unresolved mourning when treating a drug abuser. As so many more men than women become heroin addicts, this symptom may also be related to the special problems of men separating from their mothers.

Early Pregnancy As an Antidote to Hopelessness and Loss

Girls may resist separation and seek to resolve their mother's blocked grief by becoming pregnant, particularly in low-income single-parent families. As her daughter reaches puberty, the single mother, having no marital dyad in which to reinvest and few career opportunities, may fear being left alone. She may wish to keep her daughter at home or start another family. If her energies are depleted by the difficulties of living in poverty, she may not be able to renounce this wish and begin the anticipatory mourning necessary to prepare for this life transition; she may become depressed instead. The daughter may become pregnant in an attempt to avoid the feelings of loss (both hers and her mother's) that would ensue if she stayed in school, got a job, moved out, and eventually married. A baby at once binds mother and daughter together as co-parents, thus preventing their separation and providing a mutual project (Notman & Zilbach, 1975). Thus, early motherhood provides adult status for the daughter in her mother's home and protects the grandmother from the role loss that she would experience if her children grew up and left her alone.

Some women may use pregnancy to compensate for a recent or imminent death of a family member. Walsh (1978) discovered a striking concurrence of grandparent death and birth of a schizophrenic offspring. Parents were unaware of this simultaneity, but Walsh reasoned that the child may have assumed "a special replacement role" (p. 457). Similarly, Swigar, Bowers, and Fleck (1976) present seven case examples of women seeking abortion who had unintentionally become less vigilant in their usual contraceptive use in response to the death or serious illness of a parent. In her survey at two social service agencies in Michigan, Klyman (1986) noted that one-quarter of the teen-agers and almost one-half of the adult women who sought pregnancy counseling had experienced early childhood loss. She contended that preg-nancy can be a reaction to the death of a sibling in early childhood or even division of the sibling group among foster parents.

Such a dynamic can exist, of course, in middle-income families as well. The frequency of such loss is greater in the lower income groups, however. Life expectancy is lower overall. Homicide as the leading cause of death begins for black males at age 15 and continues until age 34. (Health Hazard Appraisal, 1972). More people die in each life cycle stage. Black infants die at a high rate compared to other western nations. In 1978, the Black infant mortality rate was "86% higher than the white rate . . . and essentially twice as high in 1982. While the white infant mortality rate declined by 4% in 1982, the black rate rose 2%" (Sidel, 1986).

Finally, as mentioned earlier, low-income girls may become pregnant when they are very young out of hopelessness (MacDonald, 1970). Faced with dangerous and inadequate schools and few employment opportunities if they do complete their schooling, low-income girls may find it difficult to generate the hope for a better future that would give them a reason to delay pregnancy. Feeling that their lives are primarily in the control of environmental forces, they may welcome pregnancy and the prospect of child-rearing as a way of having something of their own (Bucholz & Gol, 1986).

FAMILY REACTION TO SEXUAL ABUSE

In reviewing the debate whether sexual abuse is more prevalent in low-income groups, Parker and Parker (1986) find that "stepfathers and other father-surrogates are over-represented among abusers" (p. 533). Such abuse does appear to be very common, especially in the population served by mental health clinics. Runtz and Briere (1986) found that 15% of female college students reported one or more incidents of childhood sexual abuse, while 44% of women attending a mental health clinic reported such incidents (Briere & Runtz, in press).

A victim's reaction to sexual abuse, particularly incest, is similar to grief in several ways. The abuse is a loss of self-determination or control over personal boundaries. It is followed by painful affect, obsessive rumination, guilt, attempts to master actively what was inflicted passively, and reproachful anger. Reactions may also include the severe loss of self-esteem that is part of depression. The psychic effects can be especially devastating in the case of incest, because the victim suffered at the hands of a trusted family member. Thus, incest is not only a violation of the child's body, but a betrayal of a relationship. As a result of such an experience, the victim is likely to doubt the potential of others in the family (e.g., her mother) to protect her. This effect is seriously compounded if the victim tries to reveal the abuse to other potential protectors in or out of the family and is pressured by family members to remain silent (Sgroi, 1982). Thus, sexual abuse occasions not only the loss of personal boundaries and the loss of a trusting relationship with the abuser, but also the loss of the victim's connection to the whole family as a protective network.

Just as sexual abuse resembles loss in its effect, the process necessary for recovery from it resembles mourning: a painful, lengthy, and repeated renunciation of the compromised aspects of the relationship with the abuser. As the victim withdraws her emotional investment from the compromised relationship, she must establish a new individuated self. At this point, as in the resolution of mourning, the victim may be able to turn back toward the world and reinvest her repossessed energy in new relationships. The process of gradual and painful renunciation and reinvestment is a difficult and demanding psychic one, even for an adult. A young child may not be able to complete it because of age-appropriate immaturity. Although most mourning theorists believe that the child's ability to mourn develops with age, Wolfenstein (1966) contended that it is not until the child has had a psychically successful adolescence that the personality can support such a process.

This process can be inhibited if the family is unresponsive and, enjoins the victim to secrecy in order to preserve the family structure or, worst of all, colludes in the continuation of the abuse. These family reactions make it nearly impossible for the victim to resolve the trauma in a psychologically healthy manner. Some pathological resolution (e.g., defensive detachment, serious depression, compulsive precocious sexual activity, attempts at reenactment, or lack of sexual desire in adult life) is likely to occur.

Adult victims of childhood incest are often depressed, especially if the incest was never discovered or it was discovered and their mothers did not defend them. Such a process may have occurred in each generation of the family. The lasting effects of such trauma are not due just to the incest itself, but to the isolation of the victim from the rest of the family and the consequent inability to complete the mourning process.

RECOMMENDATIONS FOR TREATMENT

There are two common technical difficulties in therapy with low-income families:

1. When an early interview reveals a history of loss in a family, the therapist often takes "helping the family to mourn" as the primary and immediate goal.
2. The therapist sometimes attempts to reinforce the parental hierarchy— "empower" the single mother—before determining who else may be included in the network's executive subsystem.

The therapist who approaches mourning issues early in therapy may assume that the family has not mourned solely because it is fearful of painful affect. Therefore, the therapist feels that supportive confrontation of this issue will help the family overcome its fear, that a catharsis will ensue, and that the symptoms will disappear once the blocked affect is released. In some families, this approach is successful. In other families, however, this approach is unsuccessful, because unresolved mourning is only one of several problems with which the family is struggling. For these families, prematurely focusing the therapy on mourning often results in several vague and directionless sessions that do little to relieve the symptoms. Sometimes, the family leaves treatment, fleeing the painful task that has been suggested before the family has the structure to bear it.

Even in families with very obvious losses, the timing of any effort to deal with mourning is important to the success of the therapy. Structural Family Therapy techniques of *joining* and *framing* should precede any attempts to enact the mourning process (Fulmer, 1983). *Boundary-making* and *restructuring,* in that order, should then be integrated into the mourning process so as to ameliorate the family dysfunction that blocked the mourning in the first place.

The work of Doherty and Colangelo (1984) has permitted a refinement of this theory. Using the framework of Schutz's FIRO theory (1958), they contend that family therapy should deal with a family's problems in a certain order: (1) issues of membership, (2) issues of power and responsibility, and (3) issues of intimacy. They are especially emphatic that therapists should adhere to this order in the treatment of multiproblem families. In applying this formulation to therapy for low-income families, the therapist should first discover who is influential in the kinship network and what the concrete needs of the family are; if some necessary resources (either familial, material, or service) are missing, the therapist should focus on obtaining these resources. These should be considered membership issues. Then, the therapist should focus on the power relationships between members of this network. Only when these issues are resolved, should issues of intimacy (e.g., mourning) be approached.

Issues of Membership: Discovering the Kinship Network

In order to understand the context in which the low-income single mother is functioning, the therapist must determine the membership and current lines of influence in the mother's kinship network. It is especially important to determine who helps the mother to raise her children and whether anyone else has a right to comment on the mother's child-rearing practices. In addition, the therapist should ask about past changes in membership of the kinship network through death, institutional placement, and relocation. The histories of both the mother and her children may include several changes in residence, which, of course, involve separations from siblings and care-givers. Such "residence life histories" (Stack, 1974) may reveal significant losses through separation that have gone unrecognized and, so, unmourned.

While a mother's residence life history is always revealing about her past, a broader inquiry into her current extended family may reveal that she is not really in conflict with her family members. She may be truly isolated from her kin, receiving neither support nor criticism from them. For example, Martin and Martin (1978) contended that many kinship networks work well in rural settings, but deteriorate when subjected to urban environmental and public policy pressures. Rogler and his associates (1983) also speculated that "traditional bonds are also attenuated" (p. 24) for Puerto Rican families in New York City.

If the kinship network has disintegrated to the point that it can neither help nor hinder the mother, the therapist should connect the family to social agencies that provide the needed services (e.g., secure housing, food stamps, training programs, a homemaker, care for the elderly, or day care for the children). Such assistance can be a powerful joining maneuver. The therapist may also attempt to connect the mother to other parents with children of the same age, thus constructing a social network of peers (Douglas & Jason, 1986). The goal, of course, is not simply to secure specific direct services for the family; it is to unburden the mother sufficiently so that she can consistently offer guidance, support, and discipline to her children, thus restoring the organization of the family (Aponte, 1986).

Issues of Power: Clarifying the Executive Hierarchy

The inquiry may, however, reveal an intact network that could offer support to the mother. If she is not receiving it, she may be in considerable conflict with other network executives, such as her own mother, her ex-husband, her ex–mother-in-law, her sisters, or even her own adult children. The mother may not be the only "mother" of her children; she may not even be the superior or equal to all of her children's various care-givers. As in any family, different care-givers may have different rules, a situation that always creates problems. The executive subsystem of the extended family may include a "dominant figure" (Martin & Martin, 1978), without whose cooperation the family therapy will not be successful. Thus, inquiry into the executive hierarchy may be essential in discovering who in the family must be convened.

Further inquiry (through questioning or observation) into the dynamics of the network hierarchy may be necessary. For example, not all executive subsystems pertain to all the mother's children. Because of the sequence of fathers and occasional periods of informal fosterage that are common in low-income families, different groups of adults and older siblings may have acquired disciplinary rights over different children of the same mother. A mother may feel secure in her authority over certain of her children, but have to answer to another executive when she disciplines others. Thus, a mother's apparent passivity or being overwhelmed by environmental pressures may be a product of executive conflict.

If the kinship network is disabled by conflict, the therapist should proceed as if the family were a blended family, convening different groups of executives as needed and clarifying who is in charge of whom at what times, who needs help separating from whom, and who must ally with whom for the limited purpose of child-rearing (McGoldrick & Carter, 1980). The main difference between a kinship network and a blended family is that a kinship network involves three generations, sometimes creating a differentiated hierarchy *within* the "parental" subsystem. The main goal of therapy is to empower the mother by securing her place of authority with the other executives.

Discovering a Type of Hidden Conflict. Occasionally, a mother appears to have no kinship network, but is unable to use the therapist's concrete support. She consistently fails to keep appointments with social service agencies, refuses to let a hard-won homemaker enter her apartment, or precipitously withdraws her child from an adequate day care situation that she herself requested. Sometimes a mother who behaves in this manner has a reasonably intact kinship network that could provide support but is disconnected from it because of emotional conflicts and long-held grudges on both sides. Her apparent isolation is really a case of protracted executive conflict. In such cases, the harder the therapist works to make services available to her, the less the mother takes advantage of them.

For this mother, the therapist cannot simply make connections with agencies or help to reconstruct a peer network. The therapist should attempt to persuade the mother that some of her difficulties with children, agencies, and (now) the therapist are a replication of the bitter standoffs she maintains with her family of origin. If she accepts this idea (a long shot), the therapist may use Bowenian "coaching" techniques (Carter & Orfanidis, 1976) to heal the splits. This not only may free the mother's energy for present tasks, but also may reconnect her with relatives who can offer concrete assistance. If reconnection is impossible, the therapist should at least describe the repetitive pattern and make each act of further therapeutic assistance contingent on the patient's completion of a reasonable task that requires her active initiative.

Assessing Underorganization. Low-income families often appear chaotic. An apparently overwhelmed single mother may attend a therapy session with a large group of her children, her grandchildren, and even a friend's children, seeming barely in control of herself or them. Aponte (1986) described such families as "underorganized." He contended that, although family conflict is commonly considered the source of symptoms in these families, they are *not* in conflict. He stated that the level of family organization must be considered a separate source of difficulty. A similar phenomenon has been noted by Goldner (1982) in symptomatic early stage stepfamilies in which the marital pair is not in conflict, but the organization of the larger system (i.e., children, stepchildren, parents, step-parents, and ex-spouses) has not yet developed an identity.

Aponte makes a valid point when he says that underorganization is not limited to low-income families, but neither is conflict limited to middle-income families. A functioning kinship network can meet Aponte's standards of number, complexity, coherence, and continuity, and therefore, be highly organized. But the executives of any sophisticated organization can be in conflict and, thereby, impair its function. Whether a clinician sees a given family as underorganized or in conflict will have important clinical consequences.

If the therapist has searched the kinship network and ruled out the presence of hidden or overt executive conflict, the family may indeed be truly underorganized in response to environmental stress or delayed maturation. The therapist can ameliorate the underorganization temporarily by supporting the overburdened executive and helping her to secure material and social service resources. The therapist can then help differentiate roles and establish a hierarchy in the family. If the family has been organized solely by the activity and presence of the solitary executive, rules can be made and authority delegated. By this means, the executive may be unburdened, but coaching may be necessary to accomplish the dispersion of responsibility.

Issues of Intimacy: Restoring a Receptive Intimate Context

Often, an extended period of demoralization or conflict has seriously damaged the ability of family members to enjoy each other, share personal thoughts and feelings, or exchange advice or assistance. By whatever technique, a major goal of restoring an isolated, disconnected, embattled, or overburdened mother's power in the family is to permit greater intimacy between her and kin, friends, and children. An effective executive must assert hierarchical authority, but cannot influence her family by that authority alone. Her children and other kin must want to please her, show loyalty, be like her, identify themselves with family values by their behaviors, and take pleasure in exchanging emotional and concrete acts of support. These benign and intimate connections, not solely hierarchy and discipline, are what hold intimate organizations together and "empower" mothers.

"Power" in this case is ability—the ability to meet one's needs by engaging in give-and-take with others, rather than by dominating them. Positive mutual exchanges are by far the most efficient means of creating an orderly and predictable organization and will greatly decrease the mother's sense of helplessness.

As mentioned earlier, Brown and Harris (1978) found that women were more often depressed and hopeless when they lacked a "confiding" relationship with a husband or boyfriend. It is important to note that the *quality* of the relationship was the crucial factor in preventing hopelessness. Lindblad-Goldberg and Dukes (1985) reported a similar finding in a comparison of single Black mothers of dysfunctional families with single Black mothers of functional families. Both groups reported support networks of approximately the same size, but the mothers whose children had symptoms reported that their networks were not fully reciprocal; these mothers felt that they gave to others, but did not receive in kind. Again, the quality—not the quantity—of the supportive relationships appears to be the symptom-preventing factor.

Therapy for Unresolved Mourning

Clarifying kinship network membership, securing resources, and negotiating power relationships should help to relieve the hopelessness that inhibits mourning. When a sense of hopefulness and the ability to effect change are restored, mourning sometimes begins spontaneously with the mother reminiscing about her past. It may be necessary, however, to link the family symptoms explicitly to reactions to loss. Such interpretations make the pursuit of the unresolved mourning a meaningful, practical activity.

Even if the therapist does not use explicit interventions, it is important to have a theory that links the family's symptom to the unresolved mourning in a specific way. In addition to linking the unresolved feelings about a specific loss to depressed behavior, such a theory should contain at least two descriptions of interaction: (1) how the children are behaving in relation to the mother's depression and (2) how the mother can help them abandon their pathological attempts to rescue her. Such a formulation gives the mourning an interactive purpose and, therefore, gives the family therapy a direction.

If the mother accepts the therapist's invitation, mourning work may include talking over memories of the lost person, particularly the events and feelings surrounding the death; looking with the therapist at family pictures that include the deceased; or assigning the patient to interview (or bring into session) other family members who knew the deceased. Writing letters or making audiotapes for the deceased is especially useful for reworking unresolved conflicts. At first, these letters may be written or tapes recorded as if they were simply updates for the dead person about current news. Later, they should acknowledge the death and say goodbye (J. Rolland, personal communication, 1986). Stressor videotapes (Paul, 1976), graveside visits (Paul, 1967), and family-designed farewell rituals (Bowen, 1978) all may be used to conclude the mourning.

Once the mother has overcome her resistance to the mourning (even if she has not completed it), she can shift her attention to providing a receptive context for her children's concerns. They may need simply her reassurance that, although she was once unhappy, she has now recovered. If she has not recovered, she can at least reassure her children that she has help and does not need theirs.

If the children have not mourned their own losses, it may be necessary to sensitize the mother about those losses. Special attention should be given to the loss of care-givers, siblings, fathers, or even familiar residences. Ideally, the mother then acknowledges her children's unhappiness and tells them that she is willing to listen to their feelings. The therapist must advise some mothers that they should not take their children's regrets as literal requests to return to the home that they are mourning; children may be reluctant to mourn if they think their mother will try to send them back.

In helping the children, the mother may initiate talks, look over pictures with the children, share memories, or take the children for their own graveside visits. This may require considerable selflessness from the mother and is not an easy psychic task. Therefore, it is best if at least some of these interactions take place during therapy sessions so that the mother will have the therapist's support. If the family prefers to do them at home, the mother may require coaching to avoid being defensive about her role (real or imagined) in the children's loss and to realize that she need only acknowledge the children's losses sympathetically, not make them feel better. Children vary in their ability to sustain such discussions according to their age and relationship to the deceased, but it should help them to know that their mother is accessible on the subject.

Even if unresolved mourning is a partial cause for many of the symptoms manifested in family members, mourning alone is rarely enough to relieve them. All these symptoms have multiple causes and, once established, develop an autonomy such that they cannot be reversed simply by removing the causes. Thus, depression may require medication. Collusive mischief and delinquency need the restoration of a consistent hierarchy. Prevention of pregnancy requires discussion of sexual activity and the institution of a birth control regimen. Drug addiction requires careful detoxification and long-term involvement in treatment groups. Recovery from incest may be hastened by participation in survivors' groups, as well as family and individual therapy focused on that issue. In addition to these therapies, it is worthwhile to attempt to restore the family's mourning process. This will ameliorate the environment that was originally conducive to the symptoms, inoculate the family against their recurrence, and prevent their reappearance in the next generation.

REFERENCES

Aponte, H. (1986). "If I don't get simple, I cry." *Family Process, 25*(4), 531–548.

Belle, D., Ashley, P., Dever, K., Longfellow, C., Makovsky, V., Martin, J., Mitchell, J., Saunders, E., & Zelkowitz, P. (1979). Depression and low-income, female headed families. In E. Corfman (Ed.), *Families today: A research sampler on families and children: Vol. 1* (NIMH Science Monographs 1, DHEW Publication No. ADM 79-815). Washington, DC: U.S. Government Printing Office.

Bowen, M. (1978). Family reaction to death. In *Family therapy in clinical practice* (pp. 321–335). New York: Jason Aronson.

Briere, J., & Runtz, M. (in press). Post-sexual abuse trauma: Data and implications for clinical practice. *Journal of Interpersonal Violence.*

Brown, G., & Harris, T. (1978). *Social origins of depression: A study of psychiatric disorder in women.* New York: Free Press.

Buchholz, E., & Gol, B. (1986). More than playing house: A developmental perspective on the strengths in teenage motherhood. *American Journal of Orthopsychiatry, 56*(3), 347–359.

Carter, E., & Orfanidis, M. (1976). Family therapy with one person and the family therapist's own family. In P. Guerin (Ed.), *Family therapy: Theory and practice* (pp. 193–219). New York: Gardner Press.

Children's Defense Fund. (January 1986). *Adolescent pregnancy: Whose problem is it?* Adolescent Pregnancy Prevention Clearinghouse. Washington, DC.

Coleman, S. (1980). Incomplete mourning and addict family transactions: A theory for understanding heroin abuse. In D. Lettieri (Ed.), *Theories of drug abuse* (National Institute on Drug Abuse, Research Monograph 30, DHHS Publication No. ADM 80-967). Washington, DC: U.S. Government Printing Office.

Coleman, S., Kaplan, J.D., & Downing, R. (1986). Life cycle and loss—The spiritual vacuum of heroin addiction. *Family Process, 25*(1), 5–23.

Deutsch, H. (1937). Absence of grief. *Psychoanalytic Quarterly, 6,* 12–22.

Doherty, W., & Colangelo, N. (1984). A modest proposal for organizing family treatment. *Journal of Marital and Family Therapy, 10*(1), 19–29.

Douglas, J., & Jason, L. (1986). Building social support systems through a babysitting exchange program. *American Journal of Orthopsychiatry, 56*(1), 103–108.

Fulmer, R. (1983). A structural approach to unresolved mourning in single parent family systems. *Journal of Marital and Family Therapy, 9*(3), 259–268.

Furstenberg, F. (1981). Implicating the family: Teenage parenthood and kinship involvement. In T. Ooms (Ed.), *Teenage pregnancy in a family context: Implications for policy* (pp. 131–164). Philadelphia: Temple.

Garcia-Preto, N. (1982). Puerto Rican families. In M. McGoldrick, J. Pearce & J. Giordano (Eds.), *Ethnicity and family therapy* (pp. 164–186). New York: Guilford.

Gibbs, J. (1986). Assessment of depression in urban adolescent females: Implications for early intervention strategies. *American Journal of Social Psychiatry, 6*(1), 50–56.

Goldner, V. (1982). Remarriage family: Structure, system, future. In L. Messinger (Ed.), *Therapy with remarriage families* (pp. 187–206). Rockville, MD: Aspen Publishers.

Goode, W. (1963). *World revolution and family patterns.* New York: Free Press of Glencoe.

Gutman, H. (1978). *The black family in slavery and freedom: 1750–1925.* New York: Vintage.

Health Hazard Appraisal. (1972). *Probability tables of deaths in the next ten years from specific causes.* Indianapolis, IN: Methodist Hospital of Indiana.

Hoffman, L. (1981). *Foundations of family therapy.* New York: Basic Books.

Klyman, C. (1986). Pregnancy as a reaction to early childhood sibling loss. *Journal of the American Academy of Psychoanalysis, 14*(3), 323–335.

Lindblad-Goldberg, M., & Dukes, J. (1985). Social support in black, low-income, single parent families: Normative and dysfunctional patterns. *American Journal of Orthopsychiatry, 55*(1), 42–58.

MacDonald, A.P. (1970). Internal-external locus of control and the practice of birth control. *Psychology Report, 27*, 206.

McGoldrick, M., & Carter, E. (1980). Forming a remarried family. In E. Carter & M. McGoldrick (Eds.), *The family life cycle: A framework for family therapy* (pp. 265–294). New York: Gardner.

Martin, E., & Martin, J.M. (1978). *The black extended family.* Chicago: University of Chicago Press.

Minturn, L., & Lambert, W., et al. (1964). *Mothers of six cultures.* New York: Wiley, pp. 291–292.

Notman, M.T., & Zilbach, J.J. (1975). Family aspects of nonuse of contraceptives in adolescence. In H. Hirsch (Ed.), *The family. Fourth International Congress of Psychosomatic Obstetrics and Gynecology* (pp. 213–217). Basel: Karger.

O'Connell, M., & Rogers, C. (1984). Out-of-wedlock births, premarital pregnancies and their effect on family formation and dissolution. *Family Planning Perspectives, 16*(4), 157–162.

Parker, H., & Parker, S. (1986). Father-daughter sexual abuse: An emerging perspective. *American Journal of Orthopsychiatry, 56*(4), 531–549.

Paul, N. (1967). The role of mourning and empathy in conjoint marital therapy. In G.H. Zuk & I. Boszormenyi-Nagy (Eds.), *Family therapy and disturbed families* (pp. 187–205). Palo Alto, CA: Science and Behavior Books.

Paul, N. (1976). Cross-confrontation. In P.J. Guerin (Ed.), *Family therapy: Theory and practice* (pp. 520–529). New York: Gardner Press.

Rogler, L., Cooney, R., Constantino, G., Earley, B., Grossman, B., Gurak, D., Malady, R., & Rodriguez, O. (1983). *A conceptual framework for mental health research on Hispanic populations* (Monograph No. 10). Bronx, NY: Hispanic Research Center, Fordham University.

Runtz, M., & Briere, J. (1986). Adolescent "acting-out" and childhood history of sexual abuse. *Journal of Interpersonal Violence, 1*(3), 326–333.

Schutz, W. (1958). *FIRO: A three-dimensional theory of interpersonal behavior.* New York: Holt, Rinehart and Winston. Also reprinted as *The interpersonal underworld.* Palo Alto, CA: Science and Behavior Books, 1966.

Sgroi, S. (1982). *Handbook of clinical intervention in child sexual abuse.* Lexington, MA: Lexington Books, D.C. Heath.

Stack, C.B. (1974). *All our kin: Strategies for survival in a black community.* New York: Harper.

Stanton, M.D. (1977). The addict as savior: Heroin, death and the family. *Family Process, 16*(2), 191–197.

Stanton, M.D., & Todd, T. (1982). *The family therapy of drug abuse and addiction.* New York: Guilford.

Swigar, M., Bowers, M., & Fleck, S. (1976). Grieving and unplanned pregnancy. *Psychiatry, 39*, 72–80.

Walsh, F. (1978). Concurrent grandparent death and birth of schizophrenic offspring. *Family Process, 17*(4), 457–464.

Winch, R.F., & Blumberg, R.L. (1971). Societal complexity and familial organization. In A. Skolnick & J. Skolnick (Eds.), *Family in transition* (pp. 122–144). Boston: Little, Brown.

Wolfenstein, M. (1966). How is mourning possible? *Psychoanalytic Study of the Child, 21*, 93–123.

3. The Assessment of Social Networks in Black, Low-Income Single-Parent Families

Marion Lindblad-Goldberg, PhD
Associate Clinical Professor of Psychology in the Department of Psychiatry
University of Pennsylvania
and
Director, Family Therapy Training Center
Philadelphia Child Guidance Clinic
Philadelphia, Pennsylvania

M any authorities claim that the nuclear family is decaying as the number of single-parent households is increasing. Because the single-parent family does not conform to the ideal standard of American life in a two-parent family, these authorities (and members of the public) have often pejoratively labeled the single-parent family as "deviant," "unstable," or "disintegrated" rather than view the single-parent family as simply an alternate family form. *Low-income* single-parent families particularly have been subjected to this pejorative labeling, as evidenced by the vocabulary used to describe them in the mental health literature (e.g., "apathetic," "disorganized," "multiproblem," and "disadvantaged"). Defining this population by means of negative symbols, especially symbols that indicate deficits, has not been useful to professionals who work with these families.

Afro-American low-income single-parent families have been perhaps most vulnerable to cultural stereotypes and myths, particularly when considered in the context of American middle-class culture rather than in the context of a distinct Black cultural tradition. In research studies prior to the 1960s, investigators emphasized the nuclear family model and compared Black minority families to White majority families in terms of the majority group norms (Wilson, 1986). During the 1960s, researchers focused on the ways in which oppressed Black families adapted to negative societal conditions. Both research trends resulted in negative labeling of these families, because they were based on two incorrect assumptions: (1) Blacks comprise a homogeneous group, and (2) there is a general cultural equivalence between Black and White Americans with White middle-class norms as the common standard (Wilson, 1986). More recently, research studies on Black families have acknowledged the unique cultural traditions of this group. According to Wilson (1986), the assumptions underlying a cultural approach to understanding Black families are that

a. the origins of Black culture are tied to an African heritage that is expressed within an American context
b. the Black, ethnic minority is characterized by cultural values and beliefs that are distinct from the White majority
c. Black family structures vary according to demographic, situational, and personal parameters (p. 248)

The cultural variations in Black family form and functions are strengths rather than deficits, as they permit the family to survive under extreme economic and social conditions. For example, one of the most significant Black cultural patterns for the survival and maintenance of Black single-parent families is the use of extensive social networks. Furthermore, the single-parent family is simply an alternate family form and, like any other family, performs specific internal or external functions well or poorly in certain life situations and at given points in time. Thus, it may be more useful to the clinician to describe these families in terms of what they *do* rather than what they *are*. "Doing" occurs along a continuum; "being" either is or is not.

MODEL OF A WELL-FUNCTIONING BLACK LOW-INCOME SINGLE-PARENT FAMILY

Although Black extended single-parent families living in poverty are potentially sound family structures, there have been few descriptions of "healthy" functioning in these families. The need for a model of a well-functioning family within this population arose in the course of clinical and community work at the Philadelphia Child Guidance Clinic. Consequently, Lindblad-Goldberg and Dukes (1985) designed a research program to examine normative and symptomatic single-parent family functioning in Black, low-income, working and nonworking, female-headed families. The basic research assumption was that adaptive or nonadaptive functioning in these families would be related to (1) the use of social supports, (2) the quality and quantity of environmental stress, (3) the level of family organization, and (4) family members' internal perceptions of the family as a cohesive unit.

A total of 126 families were studied; 70 were classified as functional, and 56 were receiving treatment at the Clinic. All families were recruited according to the following criteria:

1. The single parent who lived in the home was the biological mother.
2. The single parenthood status had existed for at least 1 year.
3. At least two children between the ages of 6 and 18, one of whom was 10 or older, were living in the home.
4. No children in the family were mentally retarded, psychotic, severely physically handicapped, or chronically ill.
5. The gross family income was at or below the poverty level.

Families were accepted for study when some others were living in the home, but no family was accepted if an unrelated male care-giver lived in the home on a regular basis.

The screening procedure for identifying the 70 successfully functioning families included a telephone interview, a home interview, and an interview with the children's school counselor. Basically, the investigators sought families whose members had no history of child abuse, delinquency, alcohol or other substance abuse, poor social relations (children), criminal charges, school problems (behavioral or academic), chronic illness, physical handicaps, or use of mental health or mental retardation services. The comparison group consisted of 56 families referred to the Philadelphia Child Guidance Clinic's Outpatient Service, who agreed to participate in the research project at the time of their initial contact with the Clinic and who met the project's criteria for family eligibility. These families were called "symptomatic," because they had identified themselves as families in need of some help. The majority of these families had been self-referred to the Clinic, most frequently because a child was having behavior problems in school (e.g., fighting, stealing, poor peer relations).

Demographically, the two groups of families were quite similar (Lindblad-Goldberg & Dukes, 1985). The sample was composed of mothers who were in their early 30s and had an average of three children, including equal numbers of boys and girls, and ranging from predominantly preadolescents to adults. The groups did not differ in employment status, length of time since last job, occupational level, or educational level. The mothers in both groups were most frequently semiskilled workers with 12 years of education. Eighty percent of well-functioning families and 70% of symptomatic families had incomes below $6,000, which was far below the $10,000 poverty level as defined by the Pennsylvania Department of Public Assistance in 1979.

It was concluded after this study that the mother's social network profoundly affects family functioning (Lindblad-Goldberg & Dukes, 1985).

Therefore, a clinical assessment of Black single-parent families should include determinations of who is in the mother's social network and whether the network members enhance or inhibit optimal family functioning.

CHARACTERISTICS OF SOCIAL NETWORKS

The term *social support system* is often used generically, ambiguously, or even inaccurately. A social network is not necessarily a social support system. Social networks consist of social interactions that range from supportive to innocuous to destructive. Single mothers define their social network by indicating the people who are important in their lives, whether liked or disliked. The resulting network may include nuclear family, family of origin, relatives, friends, co-workers, or others who have instrumental and/or affective linkages to the mother (Pattison, Defrancisco, Wood, Frazier, & Crowder, 1975).

Hurd and his associates (1981) indicated that social networks have both structural and functional dimensions. Structurally, a network is composed of individuals who are connected to one another socially or behaviorally. Some of the structural features of social networks are

- size: the number of persons listed by the mother
- connectiveness: linkages between people who know each other
- compositions: the number and kind of relations contained within the network (i.e., family, relatives, friends, co-workers, others).

The functional features of a social network include

- affective functions: the frequency, amount, and quality of emotional exchange (positive or negative)
- instrumental functions: the frequency, amount, and quality of material assistance provided, required, or withheld
- reciprocity: the quality and intensity of obligation incurred or required as a result of giving or receiving in an instrumental or affective exchange

According to Malson (1983), the participation of Black families in mutual exchange systems is based on (1) the Afro-American tradition of doing for others, (2) the need for economic support, and (3) the functional network of support systems and the services provided. Implicit in all these is the concept that there are certain understandings between persons who participate in an exchange. Stack (1974) termed these understandings "reciprocity." McAdoo

(1979) referred to this process as "kin insurance," that is, persons whom one provides for today can be counted on tomorrow.

ASSESSMENT OF SINGLE MOTHERS' SOCIAL NETWORKS

Clinicians can assess both the structural and functional dimensions of a single mother's social network by asking questions adapted from Pattison et al. (1975) Psychosocial Inventory.

Structural Dimension

In assessing the structural dimension of a single mother's social network, the clinician may ask the mother

1. who are the subjectively important people in her life under the categories of family, relatives, friends, co-workers, and others
2. if any of these people are important because the mother does not like them or because they create problems
3. if any one of these people is dead, but remains important to the mother
4. what are the age, sex, and level of emotional importance (i.e., most, average, least) of each network member, and how long the mother has known each
5. how often (e.g., daily, once a week or month, every 6 months, once a year) the mother has contact with each network member face to face, by telephone, or by letter
6. how close the network member lives to the mother
7. what formal or informal community associations (e.g., church, social service agencies) does the mother belong to

The size of social networks for well-functioning and symptomatic families in the study at the Philadelphia Child Guidance Clinic was similar. Both groups had small networks of 12 persons who were 2 to 4 years older than the mother and whom the mother had known since she was a teen-ager. The mothers perceived their immediate family as the largest component of their network, but they also included friends and relatives. The most frequently named network categories for both groups were, in order, family (i.e., the mothers' biological and other children, ex-spouses, the mothers' siblings, and the mothers' parent[s]; friends (both female and male); and relatives (i.e., aunts, uncles, female and male cousins, nieces, nephews, and in-laws). Many network members knew each other.

In comparison to mothers in adaptive families, mothers in symptomatic families more frequently included biological children who no longer lived at home and also spontaneously mentioned people who were deceased as important network persons. These mothers' inability to detach from children in the process of separation from the family and the maintenance of ties to deceased network members may result from unresolved mourning and/or difficulty in developing new resources in a network.

Mothers in symptomatic families more frequently reported the importance of boyfriends or fiancès in their networks. Examination of the family therapy clinical records of these families revealed that problems were always evident in the relationships of the mother, the identified patient, and the boyfriend/fiancè.

The frequency of contact with and the physical distance from family and friends was similar for both groups. Mothers in symptomatic families tended to have more frequent contact with relatives and lived closer to them than did mothers in adaptive families, however.

While the well-functioning and symptomatic families did not differ in the numbers of community associations they belonged to (Lindblad-Goldberg & Dukes, 1985), membership in community organizations was related to positive perception of potentially stressful life events (Lindblad-Goldberg, Dukes, & Lasley, in press).

Functional Dimension

In assessing the functional dimension of a single mother's social network, the clinician may investigate affective and instrumental functions by asking the mother

1. what positive, negative, or mixed feelings or thoughts the mother has toward each network person
2. how intense (i.e., strong, moderate, weak) her feelings or thoughts are toward each network person
3. how frequently (i.e., often, sometimes, never) the mother helps each network person by providing emotional support when he or she needs it in the areas of parenting, personal relationships, and work stress
4. how frequently (i.e., often, sometimes, never) the mother helps each network person by providing assistance when he or she needs it in the areas of child care, finances, material goods, and household maintenance

Both groups of single mothers in the study had positive, intense feelings about members of their social network. The two groups also did not differ in the frequency of emotional or instrumental support provided to family or friends. Mothers in symptomatic families tended to provide more frequent emotional and instrumental support to relatives than did adaptive mothers, however.

In assessing reciprocity, the clinician may ask the single mother

1. what kind of feeling (i.e., positive, negative, neutral) each network person has about the mother
2. how intense (i.e., strong, moderate, weak) are the feelings of each network person about the mother
3. how frequently (i.e., often, sometimes, never) each network person helps the mother by providing emotional support when she needs it in the areas of parenting, personal relationships, and work stress
4. how frequently (i.e., often, sometimes, never) each network person helps her by providing assistance when she needs it in the areas of child care, finances, material goods, and household maintenance

While mothers in adaptive families reported an equal balance of give-and-take regarding emotional and instrumental functions between themselves and network members, mothers in symptomatic families felt that they gave more instrumental and emotional support than they received from all network members, especially from family members. The two groups did not differ in their perceptions of the kind of feeling or strength of feeling that network members expressed toward them.

CONCLUSION

While there are many similarities in the size and composition of the social networks developed by well-functioning and symptomatic Black, low-income single-parent families, the functional nature of the network appears to be most relevant in understanding what facilitates optimal functioning in these families. When impoverished single parents enter into involuntary interdependence with others because of economic stress and when the relationship is not reciprocal, the premium paid for kin insurance may be too high. The price of these stressful social ties may be symptomatic behavior in a family member.

REFERENCES

Hurd, G., Pattison, E., & Llamas, R. (1981). Models of social network intervention. *International Journal of Family Therapy, 3,* 246–257.

Lindblad-Goldberg, M., & Dukes, J. (1985). Social support in Black, low-income, single-parent families: Normative and dysfunctional patterns. *American Journal of Orthopsychiatry, 55,* 42–58.

Lindblad-Goldberg, M., Dukes, J., & Lasley, J. (in press). Stress in Black, low-income, single-parent families: Normative and dysfunctional patterns. *American Journal of Orthopsychiatry*.

Malson, M. (1983). The social support systems of Black families. *Marriage and Family Review*, 5(4), 37–57.

McAdoo, H. (1979, May). Black kinship. *Psychology Today*, pp. 67–110.

Pattison, E.,Defrancisco, D., Wood, P., Frazier, H., & Crowder, J. (1975). A psychosocial kinship model for family therapy. *American Journal of Psychiatry, 132*, 1246–1251.

Stack, C. (1974). *All our kin*. New York: Harper.

Wilson, M. (1986). The black extended family: An analytical consideration. *Developmental Psychology, 22*, 246–258.

4. Dysfunctional Arrangements in Divorcing Families

Marla Beth Isaacs, PhD
Assistant Professor
Department of Psychiatry
School of Medicine
University of Pennsylvania
Formerly,
Director and Principal Investigator
Families of Divorce Project
Philadelphia Child Guidance Clinic
Philadelphia, Pennsylvania

The family does not die with a divorce, but rather evolves structurally into a new arrangement. An important feature of the postseparation adjustment, particularly for the children, is the nature of this new arrangement. When successful, it ensures the children of a continuing relationship with each parent. The parents are able to reach appropriate decisions on custody and visitation, as well as to negotiate support issues. Although the parents may be far from friendly with each other, they are able to contain their animosity and continue to parent their children. The two new households develop a modus vivendi.

Sometimes, however, families are unable to accomplish the necessary tasks after a separation. At one extreme, families may become fragmented and splintered, with parents no longer available to protect their children and set limits for them. At the other extreme, families may deny the separation and rigidly perpetuate old patterns that jeopardize the future development of family members.

Our model of intervention is aimed at preempting fragmentation or rigidification in order to facilitate "good enough" arrangements between parents and children (Isaacs, Montalvo, & Abelsohn, 1986). The backbone of

Note: Work on this article was supported by a grant from Pew Memorial Trust to the Families of Divorce Project at the Philadelphia Child Guidance Clinic. The author would like to thank Braulio Montalvo for his careful review of the manuscript.

these arrangements includes the children's open access to the noncustodial parent and assurance that two parents are raising them. Additionally, in arrangements that facilitate a child's adjustment, the essential care-giving dialogue between the parents continues, and any hostility between them is contained in order to keep its effect on the children at a minimum.

Although the therapist may meet with the whole family, with different constellations, or with individual members of a family at various times, the first commitment is to support the parents so that they can be responsible parents through the crisis. Separated parents often feel guilty for what they have imposed on their children, and they may feel doubly guilty when things then go poorly for their children. The ability to help their children establishes an island of self-esteem and competency to counter parents' feelings of failure. In fact, a feeling of competency in handling the children bodes well for both parents and children alike.

In planning interventions, the therapist gives particular attention to the structure of the family, the role that the child or adolescent has played in the family, and the way in which that role will now change. Alliances in the family and their probable shifts after a separation are also relevant. Finally, the therapist assesses the structure and the limit-setting, as well as the nurturance, provided by the parents.

Traditionally, therapists have approached the treatment of families in which the parents are divorcing from a developmental perspective, focusing on the child's reaction to the separation as a function of age and intrapsychic experience (Tessman, 1978; Wallerstein & Kelly, 1980). While these elements of the situation cannot be ignored, neither can the arrangement of family members around the child be overlooked. Such arrangements help to shape the child's intrapsychic reactions to the separation, and this broader context provides a more satisfactory framework for developing therapeutic strategy in short-term divorce therapy.

CAUGHT IN THE MIDDLE: DYSFUNCTIONAL STRUCTURES

When parents separate, the child can be caught in the middle between the mother and the father. The angrier that the parents are with each other, the more likely that the child will be in this predicament. The different ways in which the child may be caught in the middle represent different levels of stress and pathology. The problem can range from a youngster's manageable need to please a parent to a far less manageable state of fusion with one parent.

An Excessive Need To Please

On the most benign level, a child who is caught between divorcing parents may feel the need to please one or both parents. Although attempting to please a parent is a normal process that facilitates socialization, this process may become distorted and extremely demanding during a separation. For example, a child may severely inhibit his or her normal feelings of aggression against a parent for fear of losing that parent.

Rob, a 16-year-old boy, describes to his therapist what happens when he visits his father and then returns to his mother:

Therapist: What are some of the ways you feel in the middle?

Rob: When I go there, there are certain subjects I might agree with and not agree with, and I get static from both sides. And I don't know what to do. *I can't please one without pleasing the other.* I would really be better off really if I didn't see any of them.

In part, this is a slip of the tongue. Rob meant to say, "I cannot please one without displeasing the other." Yet, he also feels he has to "please both," a draining task.

Therapist: What would keep you out of the middle?

Rob: *Live on a desert island by myself* . . . I can't do something without hurting one, without hurting the other. Little kids, they can get out of it—they have baseball, etc. I can't. I have to give an adult answer. I have everything on me.

Rob's fantasized solution is the time-honored one of the escape from the family, but the preferred escape is the allure of regression—"Little kids, they can get out of it."

A Need To Protect (Reversal of the Hierarchy)

A more stressful arrangement is one in which the child feels a need not only to please a parent, but also to protect that parent. This extreme represents a hierarchical reversal; the child can no longer be a child, because the child's main mandate is to protect the parent.

> Trevor, aged 8, feels not only a need to please his parents, but also a need to protect his mother. He is an overtaxed youngster, raised by two adults in a skewed arrangement in which one of them, the mother, competes with the father for "more of him." Here, the child and his mother are speaking to the therapist:
>
> Trevor: On Sunday, my mom and dad were having an argument about where I should go for Easter—to my mother's or father's place. And I didn't say anything. When my father was leaving, I asked Mom, "Can I go into the other room when you and dad are arguing, cause it upsets me." She said "Yes" and "Did you tell this to your father?" I said "No." And as he was leaving, she stopped him and so (*very exasperated*) I said the same thing to him, and now I'm having trouble deciding where I'm going to stay for Easter.
>
> Mother: (*defensive and angry*): But he forgets to say, he only says these things to me.
>
> His mother is telling Trevor, "Why complain only to me!" thus implicitly asking him to be fair to her almost as a child would ask a parent. In this reversal of the hierarchy, Trevor's mother is not helping him to move away from the middle.
>
> Trevor: I'm glad it's not mixed up anymore . . . cause I thought my father would get mad if I stayed at my Mom's house, and you [mother] would get mad if I stayed at Daddy's, but you said it was

OK if I stayed there for Easter.

Therapist: It's real hard to try to be there for both of them, isn't it, Trevor?

Mother: He tries awful hard.

Therapist: I'm sure he does.

Trevor's mother is not uncomfortable with her son's predicament, but instead praises him for trying to please both parents. In a healthier arrangement, the mother would not want her child in this situation.

Therapist: Are there other ways they don't get along that upset you, Trevor?

Trevor: When they yell at each other, that upsets me, as I'm afraid he'll get so mad and hit her and if he does I'll be so mad, I'm going to "spaz" out and start swinging punches.

Therapist: And you really don't want to do that, do you?

Trevor: Could hurt someone, like when my mother's getting up from the smack, I might come around, miss her, and go "bah" (*smacking his one fist into the other*) and hit her as I come around.

Therapist: Does this really make you angry when you see them argue?

Trevor: Yeah, sometimes I think my father will hit her, and sometimes I think my mother will end up hitting, and they'll be in a war, and I'll have to break it up somehow, and if I can't . . . I have to let them be.

Therapist: That's tough to think
   about. Does it happen very
   often, that you see them
   argue?
Trevor: Only on Sun-
   days . . . that one Sunday
   when he brought me back
   they were arguing so madly.
   I felt like getting up and saying (*yelling*) "Stop it!"
Therapist: What did you do?
Trevor: I kept sitting there and
   saying, "Why is this happen-
   ing to me? Why does this
   always have to happen to
   me?"

The hopeless position of having to protect his parents from violence against each other leads only to paralysis and to philosoph-
ical self-pity, a feeling that he has been "chosen" by unknown
forces for special punishment.

Alliance with One Side against the Other

   An arrangement in which the child becomes the full-blown coalitionary
partner of a parent (i.e., a fixed ally and tool of one parent against the other) is
particularly stressful. In the worst scenario, the child becomes the weapon of
one parent, which openly jeopardizes the child's relationship with the other
parent. Although the child is ostensibly committed to one side, buried long-
ings for the other parent create consuming conflict and tension for the child.

Six-year-old Brian was brought to therapy after lunging at his
father with a kitchen knife in the midst of one of his parents'
frequent fights. This very bright child had asked to see the
therapist alone and wanted to know if the therapist could help him
with his problem.
Brian: Should I love my dad or
   hate my dad? And I can't
   stop that. I don't know if I
   should love him or hate him. I
   can't make that decision.
   Can you help me with that?

Therapist: Yes. Your question is should you love your dad or hate your dad? Why would you hate your dad?

Brian: In the first place, he argues with my mom, and I asked him to turn on the checking account and he doesn't. I really think I should hate him, but I don't want to. And I can't make the decision. I keep on promising myself that I'll make it, and I don't. I just don't.

The first order of business with this family is to help the parents see and acknowledge the toll that their behavior is having on their child and to help them separate responsibly.

Embodiment of Parental Conflict (Fusion)

One of the most stressful arrangements is that in which the child comes to embody the parental conflict.

As a result of a physical joint custody arrangement that required almost daily shifts of residence, 7-year-old Kevin had begun to show signs of deep personality impairment.

Therapist: Where do you live?

Kevin: It's a long story, cause I'm in two places. We're both divorced, Daddy and Mommy.

Kevin's comment "we're both divorced" is a sign of fusion with his parents.

The schedule with which Kevin must contend would be difficult for most adults.

Kevin: I'm with my mom Monday, Thursday, and sometimes on the weekends.

Therapist: Monday through Thursday?

Father: No, Monday and Thursday. He's with me Tuesday and Wednesday.

Therapist (*confused*): Friday
and the weekends?
Kevin: They each get 5 days.

> The child implies that the arrangement is fair and equal for each of the parents.

Father: Full weekends, that's
Friday to Monday.
Therapist: Oh, how's that
working?
Kevin (*sadly*): Good.

The parents explained to the therapist that the summer had been a difficult period because their arrangement had changed; Kevin spent half of the summer with each. Kevin's father noticed that his son was particularly distressed at the end of the summer and interpreted this as an expression of preference "for one area or the other—mine this time." In other words, he interpreted the boy's unhappiness as a desire to be with him more. The father felt that the summer arrangement caused Kevin to feel "tugs of loyalty." He decided that his son needed an advocate and entered therapy partially for this reason.

Kevin certainly did need an advocate. His parents never attended to his needs in a coordinated, responsive fashion. Instead, in an effort to be fair to each other, they used an algebraic formula to divide the time equally with their son. This overprincipled attempt to "play fair" as ex-spouses overrode their parental concern about disrupting the boy's life. The therapist ascertained that Kevin was upset at the end of the summer because a period of stability was ending, and he knew he would soon be switching back and forth between his parents again. When alone with the therapist, the child was explicit about the difficulty.

Therapist: So tell me, what's
been hard for you since your
parents separated?
Kevin: Moving back and forth!

This was a joint custody arrangement gone awry, for it turned out to be punishing and rigid for Kevin. The inherent difficulties of the transition were compounded by the fact that the mother's primary language was French, and the boy was not allowed to speak English when he was with her. During this period of constant moving, Kevin told his father that he missed him. In an effort to solve this problem, the parents agreed to an even more taxing arrangement; Kevin had to see his father for a few hours on the Sunday that he was with his mother.

Therpaist: How do you work it out, when you have to go from house to house?

Kevin: Er, place to place.

Therapist: Place to place.

Kevin: What did you just say?

> He quickly loses focus and forgets while discussing this anxiety-producing topic.

Therapist: How do you remember that this is the day?

Kevin: Cause we planned a plan, and I know the plans. I don't know why. I know what days I'm with my father, what days with my mother. What gets confusing, well not confusing, gets kind of silly, [is] when on weekends with my mother, so then my mother gives me a surprise, and I'm with my daddy for a couple of hours.

Therapist: Why did they plan that?

Kevin: My parents didn't plan that. I planned it.

Therapist: Why?

Kevin: I thought that was too much time with my mother.

> Kevin protects his parents. He first describes the situation as confusing and silly, then modifies his own criticism with the positive-sounding phrase "gives me a surprise." Kevin goes on to claim that the time with his father was his own idea. This is the ultimate defense of his parents, a basic counterreaction to his complete lack of control over the situation.

Kevin then embellishes his protective rationalization for his parents' arrangement for him.

Kevin: Boys like boys, and girls like girls. Boys get together with boys. I don't have any brothers and sisters, so my dad and me always act crazy. Not my mom, she does stuff that girls do. They calm down. Boys keep going crazy and keep laughing and . . .

Therapist: Let me ask you this. You said this was your decision to spend 2 hours with your dad on weekends, and now you're saying it's not working out well; it's silly, kind of confusing.

Kevin: Not silly.

Therapist: But confusing?

Kevin: Yeah.

Therapist: Because you start doing something with your mom, and you have to drop it to go with your dad?

Kevin: I don't drop it. I leave it in my head . . . I don't let it fly out. I have it in jail until my dad has to take me over to my mother's. You open up the gate, and it flies out of there, out of the brain.

Therapist: You put it out of your mind?

Kevin (*sadly*): I don't think I can. I don't have any gates. It goes in here (*pointing to the back of his head*) and then my mom in the weekends. I don't give any signs; it just remembers what it has to do and goes back into the brain.

Therapist: You mean your schedule?

Kevin: So when the fun is over with my dad, it goes up there (*pointing again to the back of his head*) and stays stuck there.

Kevin has no firm boundaries. His attempts to maintain continuity are shown through a distorted self-image. He perceives his head as a set of chambers with gates that he must actively and desperately control to prevent the loss of the disrupted activity—the fun that is his tie to his father.

It is the fun with the father that the child was referring to.

Therapist: So that's how you work your brain. You switch it on and off.

Kevin: I can't. It's always on. The wheels and cranks are always turning, the control of the memory. Now it's in here.

Therapist: So the way you work it out, you put it back there until the time comes?

Kevin: OK, so the cranks rewind.

Therapist: So tell me how you work it out with your brain?

Kevin: I was kinda joking, I just explained it. Illustrate on the memory so it won't fly out to someone else's head, as I won't remember. If my mom says I'm going to my dad's, I'll say, "No, no." There's no way to get it back. I need this hair (*pointing to his hair*) . . . so the memory stays in.

Kevin has some awareness (a good prognostic sign) that the obsession with the control of his mechanical brain may appear aberrant to the listener—"I was kinda joking." The inadequacy of his external boundaries leaves the internal world of his thoughts exposed. In Kevin's metaphor, he needs his hair to keep his memory. He feels transparent and vulnerable without shields or covering. Kevin's mechanical brain responds to a mechanical joint arrangement by doing all it can to conserve and preserve continuity.

As a result of the dysfunctional arrangement established by his parents, Kevin exhibits extreme cognitive confusion. He can never relax and is obsessed with the stresses that the arrangement places on him. Therapy for Kevin must address his disordered thinking by helping to strengthen his ego functions. Because he needs some sameness and stability, there must be changes in the living arrangement and the attentiveness of the parents. The first step, therefore, is to fashion a more workable joint custody arrangement.

As in other arrangements, an accurate reading of the child's distress makes it possible to work with the parents and facilitate change.

SHIFTS IN THE SIBLING SUBSYSTEM

Parent-child relationships often co-exist with collateral arrangements that involve siblings. A child can be in the middle, but a middle that is shared, or a child can take turns with a sibling in protecting a parent. A child can be in a supportive sibling subsystem that facilitates flexible access to each parent or in a nonsupportive sibling subsystem that prevents flexible access to the parents. The realignments of relationships during or after separation can place excessive stress on the sibling subsystem and necessitate therapy for the siblings.

> Although still living together at the time of therapy, 12-year-old Lana's parents planned to separate imminently. Lana was beginning to wonder how her relationships with her younger sister and with her father would change when her father left. As she was close to her mother and had acted as her mother's ally, Lana was worried that her father might make her pay for that closeness after the separation by favoring her younger sister. She expected her sister to develop an intense coalition with their father that would exclude her.
>
> Therapist: Do you feel that you would have a tough time with him and your sister? Do you feel that they're closer than you are to your dad?
>
> Lana: Well, he says he's closer to me, but I think he's closer to Maya, because she's younger and, you know, she'll listen to him. Most of the time, me and my dad disagree. I'd say, "No, I want to do this" and he's the one that gets me everything, and if, you know, I'm mean to him, he's probably going to say, "I'm not getting her anything."

Therapist: So you worry about that?

Lana: So I sort of worry, you know, that he's going to betray me or something and go to my sister and get her everything she wants, while I'll be left behind.

Therapist: Oh, so you'd like to be treated equal to Maya?

Lana: I think I am all right now, but I worry about later.

Children often worry about shifts that may occur in their relationships after a separation.

In 12-year-old Michelle's family, the parents had already separated. The mother left the home, and the father stayed behind with his four daughters. As the family composition altered, Michelle was at increasing risk of abuse by her father.

Michelle (*talking about her father*): And he just started hitting me, and he does it to me all the time.

Therapist: Do you get hurt?

Michelle: My nose was swollen.

Therapist: Is this what happens when your mom's not there?

Sister: Yes, yes. He always picks on Michelle, 'cause she favors my mom more.

Michelle lived with her father, but "belonged" to her mother. She became her father's victim because she had been left behind by her coalitionary partner, her mother. That position—living with one parent while being closer to the parent who left—is always a dangerous one.

CONCLUSION

Children locked into rigid positions of pleasing and protecting their parents, as were Rob and Trevor, need to be helped out of those positions through work with the adults who uphold the arrangement. Kevin, the child who moved back and forth and had "no gates," needed a living arrangement of greater stability and sensitivity to his needs. Twelve-year-old Lana, who was worrying about the security of her relationship with her father, needed help in preparing for the imminent separation. Lana's father needed to learn that, although his older daughter was protective of his wife, she loved him very much and wanted to be assured of a continuing relationship with him. Work with Lana's mother focused on getting her support for Lana's continued involvement with her father, despite the considerable hostility between the parents. For Michelle, who was physically abused in the "enemy camp," the initial work was designed to end the abuse and to help the parents deal more directly with each other so that Michelle's father would not perceive her as a stand-in for her mother.

These different structural arrangements were associated, in semipredictable ways, with varying degrees of stress and pathology. Some of the structures were quite harmful and stressful; others were more benign, but nonetheless painful for the children. Effective therapy in all these families was based on a careful reading of the child's position in the family; the therapist used that understanding to render feedback to the parents and effect change. Children and adolescents often speak directly of their predicament in dysfunctional arrangements and may implicitly refer to the therapeutic changes necessary to relieve or release them.

REFERENCES

Isaacs, M.B., Montalvo, B., & Abelsohn, D. (1986). *The difficult divorce: Therapy for children and families*. New York: Basic Books.

Tessman, L. (1978). *Children of parting parents*. New York: Jason Aronson.

Wallerstein, J., & Kelly J. (1980). *Surviving the breakup: How children and parents cope with divorce*. New York: Basic Books.

5. Adolescent Single-Parent Families

Jay Ann Jemail, PhD
Licensed Psychologist
Department of Psychiatry
University of Pennsylvania
Philadelphia, Pennsylvania

Madelaine Nathanson, PhD
Clinical Psychologist
Philadelphia Child Guidance Clinic and
University of Pennsylvania School of Medicine
Philadelphia, Pennsylvania

Teen-age pregnancy and the growing number of adolescents who engage in unprotected sexual intercourse are matters of great public concern. The rate of illegitimate births to teen-aged girls in the United States has increased approximately threefold in the last four decades. The pregnancy rate has increased most among those under 17 years of age. One of ten adolescent girls in the United States will become pregnant before age 17. Not only does pregnancy jeopardize the social and educational well-being and the future of the adolescent mother herself (Baldwin, 1976; Baldwin & Cain, 1981; Burchinal, 1959; Card & Wise, 1978; Christanen, 1960; Furstenberg, 1976; Trussel & Menken, 1981), but also her child is more likely to have problems with health and cognitive development than is a child born of an older mother (Baldwin & Cain, 1981; Lincoln, Jaffe & Ambrose, 1976; Nortman, 1974).

The research on adolescent pregnancy and childbearing has been conducted in a primarily individualistic framework, as if the adolescent mother and her child existed in a social-emotional vacuum. A number of authors, however, have begun to broaden the approach and to consider the effect of the presence of other family members (if not the effect of family dynamics or structure) on the adolescent and her child. Furstenberg (1976) noted that teen-aged mothers typically live with one or both parents or with another member of the family; 94% keep their babies at home. Adolescent mothers who remain in the home are more likely to return to school and ultimately receive a high school diploma. Furthermore, more of these young mothers are employed, and fewer receive welfare. The mechanism by which their nuclear family provides support to those daughters who succeed in their academic and economic careers, in their parenting, and in their heterosexual relationships is not yet adequately understood.

Clapp and Raab (1978) stated that the adolescent mother who resides within the nuclear family has financial advantages, assistance with child care, and nurturance. They also found a deterioration in the relationship between the adolescent mother and the father of the child. In fact, fewer than one in four adolescent mothers marry the father of their baby, and this number appears to be on the decline across ethnic groups.

In a study of teen-aged and older mothers in an urban, low-income community on Chicago's South Side, Kellam, Adams, Brown, and Ensinger (1980) examined the various combinations of adults present in the household. They noted that, over time, teen-aged mothers tended to become the head of single-parent households more often than did older mothers who were living with older adults initially. As single heads of their households, these mothers were often socially isolated in terms of help with child-rearing, participation in organizations, and church attendance.

THE ADOLESCENT AND FAMILY PROJECT

During the Adolescent and Family Project conducted at the Philadelphia Child Guidance Clinic, we followed two groups of adolescents and their families for 3 years. When the study began, the adolescents in one group were experiencing an unplanned pregnancy; those in the second group were not pregnant and did not become pregnant during the study. There were three observation points:

1. during the fourth to ninth month of the adolescent's pregnancy (Time 1)
2. when the adolescent's baby was approximately 11 months old (Time 2)
3. when the baby was approximately 15 to 18 months old (Time 3)

The two groups were matched on a variety of demographic and family composition variables, and they were interviewed at the same time intervals.

The sample of 83 families with an adolescent who had an unplanned pregnancy was drawn largely from urban Philadelphia neighborhoods and consisted of Black (64%) and White (36%) families. These families did not represent cases registered for treatment at the Philadelphia Child Guidance Clinic. At Time 1, the adolescent mothers were 15.3 years of age on the average. Their average highest grade completed at Time 1 was 9.6. In 47% of the cases, the adolescent's biological mother was the single head of household;

36% of the adolescents lived with both parents, and 17% lived under some other household structure. The median household income was $7,000 to $8,000.

Trained female interviewers collected detailed data in structured individual interviews with each adolescent and her parent/guardian. Several paper-and-pencil instruments were also administered to the adolescents, their parents, and other members of their households. Family group interviews were video-taped to permit a subsequent assessment of the structure and level of function for individuals, subgroups, and the family unit as a whole.

The results of these investigations suggest that the families with a pregnant adolescent went through three recognizable stages: (1) a crisis stage, (2) a honeymoon stage, and (3) a reorganization stage. During the crisis stage, the interactions of the adolescent and her family were filled with intense emotions and conflict. Families that had not been aware of the adolescent's sexual activity were forced to acknowledge it. If abortion was still possible, various family members debated whether the pregnancy should be brought to term. Other issues that emerged at this stage involved the continuation of the adolescent's schooling, the care of the baby, living arrangements, and finances. Families often had to confront family and ethnic expectations in regard to childbearing. Adolescent childbearing may not have been new to the family, but the current pregnancy frequently required the family to discuss legacies openly. Most pregnant adolescents remained with their families or closely connected to them during this crisis stage. As the time for the baby's birth approached, the family put aside the conflicts that emerged—even if they had not been resolved—and entered a honeymoon period.

The honeymoon phase generally started near the end of the second trimester and the beginning of the third trimester of the adolescent's pregnancy. During this stage, the adolescent moved closer to her nuclear family. She stayed home more often and spent less time with her friends. Family members saw her as more involved and concerned about family affairs; they described her as more affectionate and understanding. According to them, the adolescent assumed more adultlike roles. The families of pregnant adolescents identified positive changes in the family as a unit and in individual family members, and they attributed these changes to the pregnancy.

After the baby was born, the family entered a stage of reorganization. Conflicts were often centered around issues of child care (e.g., who was responsible for what and when) and the role of the adolescent mother in the family. The hopes and expectations that emerged during the honeymoon stage were tested and perhaps challenged at this time. In the family that was functioning well, the adolescent's infant or young child was the focus of nurturance and attention. In the family that was not functioning so well, family members sometimes detoured conflict through their interactions with the adolescent's baby. When the members of a dysfunctional family disagreed, for example, they might turn to the nonverbal child and ask him or her for a decision. At the reorganization stage, the adolescent mother tried to resume her peer and school activities away from the family of origin. Her family, particularly her mother, was a crucial source of support in this endeavor. Conflict arose, however, around unresolved child care issues.

The adolescent mother's ability to define her role as a parent to her child varied according to her age and according to her intellectual and emotional resources. The extent to which the adolescent mother–child subsystem developed its own interpersonal skills and transactional patterns was affected by the clarity and appropriateness of individual and generational boundaries in the family. Ambiguity in the rules about the participation of family members in child care or too much interference from other subsystems (e.g., a sister too eager to act as a parent) decreased the differentiation of the adolescent mother–child subsystem within the family system.

Like other single-parent families, teen-aged single-parent families living with their family of origin function at various levels of family organization. Ouslan (1984) interviewed the adolescent mothers in the Adolescent and Family Project, as well as their families of origin, when their children were 15 to 18 months old. Her data showed that these families were not significantly different from the families with a nonpregnant adolescent on various dimensions of Olson's circumflex model (Olson, Sprenkle, & Russell, 1978), for example, in their perceptions of family cohesion and adaptability. The adolescent mothers in the sample were not representative of all teen-aged single-parent families, because the requirements in the research protocol that each adolescent's family of origin be interviewed probably excluded the more isolated, more poorly functioning adolescents. The data showed, however, that family functioning is as balanced or as extreme as that of any other family with a teen-ager when the adolescent mother lives with her family of origin.

The frequency of contact with the baby's father generally decreases during the adolescent's pregnancy and then stabilizes after the first year postpartum. Two years after the baby's birth, more than half of the adolescent mothers in the Adolescent and Family Project had at least weekly contact with the baby's father. In these cases, the baby's father was likely to be an age peer and often lived with his own nuclear family.

Few adolescent mothers report that they had planned to get pregnant when they did, and only some admit that they had hoped to become pregnant. Nevertheless, a pregnancy is a life event with a high stress value (Holmes & Rahe, 1967), and parenthood is a process filled with new demands, problems, and rewards. An adolescent's pregnancy may force her family to reorganize at a higher level of functioning (Russell, 1980), or it may create disorganization and chaos. In the sample selected for the Adolescent and Family Project, the adolescents and their families of origin tended to return postpartum to the level at which they had been functioning prior to the pregnancy; often, there were no significant changes in family organization and structure.

ASSESSMENT AND TREATMENT PLANNING

Weltner (1986) described four different levels of family functioning, based on the definition of the family's problem and an assessment of the family's organization. He proposed that therapists plan and use intervention techniques that match the family's particular level of functioning. Clinicians who work with adolescent mothers and their families can use Weltner's guide to help these families reorganize at a higher level of functioning or at least to prevent the deterioration of their level of functioning.

Level 1

According to Weltner (1986), a family at Level 1 is struggling with the management of basic needs. If the teen-aged mother does not have adequate shelter, food, protection, and medical care; does not receive at least minimal support from her social network to meet her own basic nurturance needs; and cannot meet the basic nurturance needs of her child, the clinician must determine who in the teen-aged mother's social network has the resources to assume an executive role and meet these needs. It may be necessary to mobilize more than one person. If the infant fails to thrive, it may be necessary for the clinician to work closely with pediatricians and other medical staff.

Since the problems are all too obvious, it is important for the clinician to search for strength in the system. Teen-aged single mothers often identify female relatives (e.g., sisters, aunts, grandmothers) as sources of support. The adolescent's own mother is the most frequently mentioned source of support. In our research, a low level of positive support from the baby's father was related to a high level of positive support from the adolescent mother's sisters. Although the adolescent mother's nuclear family provides the highest level of support, the baby's father and his family can be marshalled to provide assistance with child care.

When family support is not available, the clinician must find other supportive resources, such as friends, agencies, or community helpers. The therapist's role should be that of "convener, advocate, teacher, role model" (Weltner, 1986, p. 53). In some cases, the adolescent mother and her baby may need shelter in a social welfare agency until available supports in her own social network are evaluated and mobilized.

Level 2

Although the family at Level 2 can meet basic needs, the family is unable to provide minimal structure, limits, and safety. Again, the therapist who is working on the problems should focus on the family's strengths. Weltner (1986) suggested that the clinician organize those in charge and clarify expectations. Interventions may include written contracts that delegate specific tasks to each family member and built-in reinforcers.

When working with a teen-aged single-parent family functioning at Level 2, the clinician should assess the adolescent's developmental level. Parenting disrupts the normal life course of the adolescent. It can affect the adolescent mother's socialization with peers, keep her from finishing school, and, thus, limit her job opportunities. An important part of the assessment focuses on the adolescent herself. At what level was she functioning intellectually, emotionally, and socially prior to the pregnancy? What developmental tasks have been interrupted? The therapist should plan interventions that provide structure, limits, and safety for the child and allow the mother to continue her education and socialize with peers. Written contracts can help clarify the responsibilities of the individuals involved. Since repeated pregnancies are common, the therapist should discuss effective contraceptive practices with the adolescent.

The clinician needs to be innovative in order to combat the association between parenthood and adult social status in the larger cultural context. Many teen-aged mothers hope for the intrinsic rewards that parenthood brings and/or seek to acquire the status that parenthood can provide in their family and social context. Most, however, enter parenthood unaware of the sacrifices and demands that it entails. It is a challenge for clinicians who work with a teen-aged single-parent family to help them reorganize at a higher level of functioning so that the adolescent mother can eventually reap the rewards of parenthood.

Level 3

A family functioning at Level 3 is able to provide basic needs, nurturance, structure, limits, and safety. The therapeutic issues generally involve blurred or rigidly defined family, individual, and generational boundaries. It appeared that most teen-aged single-parent families in the Adolescent and Family Project had been functioning at this level prior to the pregnancy and had reorganized at this level after the birth of the child. The adolescent's child was well cared for and seemed to be thriving in the family environment. The new family member was incorporated into the structure without much, if any, reorganization or change across subsystems. In one family, for example, the adolescent's child was incorporated into the sibling subsystem, and the mother gained little special status.

> In another family, financial support was considered a requirement of parenthood. The adolescent mother and her child continued to live with her mother. Conflict arose because the mother's family objected to her maintaining a relationship with the baby's father and even to his seeing the baby since he didn't provide any financial support. Neither the adolescent mother nor the baby's father was in a position to challenge and resolve this issue. She needed her mother's assistance with child care, as well as her mother's emotional and financial support. It was predicted that, when this teen-aged single parent was in a position to separate from her mother, the level of conflict would increase.

Families at Level 3 generally resist suggestions that they enter therapy. When the task of separating from the family of origin has been a difficult task across generations, the clinician can expect even more resistance. These teen-aged single-parent families may not seek therapy until much later, perhaps not until the adolescent's child has reached adolescence.

Therapeutic strategies for Level 3 families involve the clarification of "ideal" family structure, based on ethnic and family values; they should particularly promote clarity between generations. Weltner (1986) suggested the following therapeutic techniques:

- defend family and individual boundaries
- balance triangles
- rebuild alliances
- develop generational boundaries
- assign tasks

Level 4

Although the therapist working with a family at Levels 1, 2, or 3 may touch on memories, feelings, and thoughts, they cannot be the focus of therapy. With a family at Level 4, however, the therapist concentrates on these issues. The goals are (1) to develop insight, (2) to work on self-actualization, (3) to understand legacies, (4) to clarify issues of self, and (5) to resolve problems of intimacy. The clinician can employ more traditional techniques (e.g., psychodynamic, existential approaches), either with the individual or with a group of family members.

Teen-aged single-parent families at Level 4 rarely enter treatment, perhaps because parenthood can be extremely taxing to the adolescent mother and her family. The need for therapy may not be clear until much later in life, or it may receive a low priority from generations still coping with the daily socioeconomic burdens and legacies of adolescent parenthood.

CASE EXAMPLE

Charlene, a 14-year-old Black adolescent, and her family enrolled in the Adolescent and Family Project when she was in the eighth month of her pregnancy. At that time, the household included Charlene, her mother Mrs. P. (aged 44), and her four sisters: Cheryl (aged 19), Karen (aged 18), Stephanie (aged 16), and Beverly (aged 8). An urban Philadelphia family with an annual income between $5,500 and $7,500, the family lived in a two-bedroom apartment. Mrs. P. and her husband had been separated for 6 years. At the time of the family's enrollment in the Project, Mr. P. was living in a nursing home, but he had contact with his daughters.

Charlene began engaging in sexual intercourse at age 13; the baby's father was her only partner. Neither she nor he ever used any method of contraception. Moreover, Charlene did not know the time of the menstrual cycle at which a woman was most likely to become pregnant if no contraception was used. A ninth grader, she had never had a class in which contraception was discussed, and Mrs. P. said that she and Charlene had never discussed sexual intercourse, contraception, or guidelines for what is "right and wrong" in terms of sexual behavior.

Throughout her 2-year involvement with the Project, Charlene continued her sexual relationship with the baby's father. Although Charlene used oral contraceptives in the first year after delivery, she reported that she was no longer using contraceptives 1 year later. Charlene's relationship with the baby's father and his frequent contact with the baby created conflict within her family, particularly in Charlene's interactions with her mother and Stephanie. Mrs. P. wanted the baby's father to have no contact with Charlene or the baby. Among other things, she stated that he had punched Charlene on several occasions, and Charlene herself rated her satisfaction with the relationship at only 50%, saying "Things aren't going the way I want them to."

A review of the interview data and videotapes of family group interactions indicated that the constellation of strengths and weaknesses in this family were characteristic of Level 2 functioning as described by Weltner (1986). Basic issues of nurturance and safety were handled adequately, and—despite the significant discord among some family members—minimal needs for shelter, food, clothing, medical care, and education were clearly met. The executive and sibling subsystems were blurred, however, so that certain features of adjustment were in jeopardy. Charlene, for example, was at serious risk for another pregnancy and was not progressing in school. When seen 1 year after delivery, she had been suspended from school for the remainder of the academic year because of fighting, and 1 year later had completed only tenth grade.

A great deal of open hostility between Charlene and her sister Stephanie was evident at each point of contact with the Project. It appeared that the birth of Charlene's baby had exacerbated a preexisting conflict. Stephanie fought with peers outside the home as well. In addition, it appeared to all observers of this family that the 18-year-old sister Karen was notably depressed, sitting silent and unincluded during much of the family interaction.

In violation of the age hierarchy of the siblings, Stephanie played a role in the executive system of this family. As Mrs. P.'s ally, Stephanie was often directly at odds with Charlene. In a very dramatic demonstration of Mrs. P.'s inclusion of Stephanie in the executive system, Stephanie literally functioned as her mother's mouthpiece in one task. When the family was asked to discuss as a group and decide on a single menu for a family dinner, Mrs. P. whispered her ideas and decisions to Stephanie, who in turn announced them verbatim to the family group. At the outset, Charlene's meal choices were supported by at least one other sister, but Charlene was unable to parlay this initial strength in numbers into the ultimate family choice. Seemingly unaware of her potential power in the group, she capitulated to the suggestions of her mother and Stephanie without any attempt to persuade or influence them.

Neither the pregnancy nor the birth appeared to change the structure of the executive system or to confer any special positive status on Charlene. When the clinician asked the family to discuss a recent family argument, Stephanie began the interchange by criticizing the way that Charlene dealt with the baby's dirty diapers. Very quickly, others added their critical comments, thereby joining the power coalition and undermining Charlene in her parental role.

Charlene's baby was well cared for and obviously handled by all with warmth and tenderness. Charlene and the baby were not differentiated as a distinct subsystem in any meaningful way, however. Instead, the baby had been assimilated into the sibling subsystem and was treated much like Charlene's peer. During one of the family interviews, Charlene several times attempted to exert some decision-making power over the baby by placing her in the playpen. Repeatedly, Stephanie sabotaged Charlene's efforts to assume an executive position by almost immediately removing the baby from the playpen. During a period of free play, Stephanie was very competitive and possessive in play with the baby; again, Charlene's response was a passive withdrawal.

Although the family members' basic needs were being met and the baby was being nurtured by their combined efforts, family members were experiencing distress. Charlene stated at various times that she was not happy with her relationships with her sisters and her boyfriend. When asked approximately 2 years after delivery how she would advise a teen-ager who became pregnant at the age she herself had become pregnant, Charlene responded, "First, get an abortion; second, go to a family planning clinic." Stephanie had problems with peer relationships, and Mrs. P. was feeling personally burdened and worried about her daughters. She stated,

> I haven't noticed any changes in Charlene since the baby was born. I expected things would be different. She is still the same little girl . . . did not mature any . . . sisters take care of the baby most. I don't have much time for myself. All my kids except Cheryl [the 19-year-old who moved out the house after the baby's birth] seem like they're not maturing. Any goals I had are set back.

Therapeutic interventions with this family would focus on realigning the subsystems so that Mrs. P. would function as primary family executive in her role as a mother and as a kind of advisor/consultant in her role as a grand-mother. She would not be denied assistance, as her daughters could each be enlisted for particular, specific functions. In addition, the therapist would explore the possibility of recruiting other adults in the network to provide support to Mrs. P. Releasing Stephanie from her regular position in the executive subsystem would free her to receive a different kind of leadership and guidance from her mother, which potentially could help her with her own social problems. Furthermore, by joining her siblings in an equal status position, she might begin to enjoy a sisterly camaraderie that had clearly been denied her. Again, success in her sibling group might generalize to success with peers outside the home.

The therapist would encourage Mrs. P., in her executive capacity, to bolster Charlene's specific identification as mother to the baby. Mrs. P. would probably be eager to do so if the therapist defined it as a way to help her daughter mature. Charlene's acceptance of responsibility in this area would pave the way to more responsible behavior in other areas, such as school and sexual activity. In addition, by making the effort to support Charlene's parental role, Mrs. P. would ultimately avoid the long-term implications of rearing yet another child herself, particularly at a time when she would probably like to concentrate on some of her own goals.

In attempting to effect such family restructuring, the therapist would have to explain interventions as ways to fine-tune strengths already present in the system. The therapist would have to make the benefits of such changes clear to family members, particularly to Stephanie, who might resent the loss of status that she would experience if she were no longer mother's exclusive executive partner. The therapist would have to persuade Mrs. P. that her burdens would not be increased if she assumed primarily a solo parental role. Charlene would need coaching and active support to emerge from her position of passivity. As is characteristic generally of Level 2 interventions, it would be continually necessary to emphasize family strengths and successes during the restructuring process.

REFERENCES

Baldwin, W.H. (1976). Adolescent pregnancy and childbearing: Growing concerns for Americans. *Population Bulletin, 31*(2).

Baldwin, W., & Cain, V.S. (1981). The children of teenage parents. In F.F. Furstenberg, Jr., R. Lincoln, & J. Menken (Eds.), *Teenage sexuality, pregnancy and childbearing*. Philadelphia: University of Pennsylvania Press.

Burchinal, L. (1959). Adolescent role deprivation and high school age marriage. *Marriage and Family Living , 21*(4), 373–377.

Card, J.J., & Wise, L.L. (1978). Teenage mothers and teenage fathers: The impact of early childbearing on the parents' personal and professional lives. *Family Planning Perspectives, 10*(4), 199–234.

Christanen, H. (1960). Cultural relativism and premarital sex norms. *American Sociological Review, 25*, 31–39.

Clapp, D.F., & Raab, R.S. (1978). Follow up of unmarried adolescent mothers. *Social Work, 23*, 149–153.

Furstenberg, F.F., Jr. (1976). *Unplanned parenthood: The social consequences of teenage childbearing*. New York: Free Press.

Holmes, T.H., & Rahe, R.H. (1967). The social readjustment scale. *Journal of Psychosomatic Research, 11*, 213.

Kellam, S.G., Adams, R.G., Brown, C.H., & Ensinger, M.E. (1980). *The long term evolution of the family structure of teenage and older mothers* (NICHD Contract No. 1-HD-728321).

Lincoln, R., Jaffe, F.S., & Ambrose, A. (1976). *11 Million Teenagers*. New York: Alan Guttmacher Institute.

Nortman, D. (1974). Parental age as a factor in pregnancy outcome and child development. *Reports on Population Family Planning* (No. 16). New York: The Population Council.

Olson, D.H., Sprenkle, D.H., & Russell, C.S. (1978). Circumflex model of marital and family systems: I. Cohesion and adaptability dimensions, family types, and clinical applications. *Family Process, 17*, 3–27.

Ouslan, A.M. (1984). *Adolescent pregnancy and parenthood: Effects on family cohesion and adaptability*. Unpublished doctoral dissertation, Temple University, Philadelphia.

Russell, C.S. (1980). Unscheduled parenthood: Transition to parent for the teenager. *Journal of Social Issues, 36*(1), 45–63.

Trussell, J., & Manken, J. (1981). Early childbearing and subsequent fertility. In F.F. Furstenberg, Jr., R. Lincoln, & J. Menken (Eds.), *Teenage sexuality, pregnancy, and childbearing*. Philadelphia: University of Pennsylvania Press.

Weltner, J.S. (1986). A matchmaker's guide to family therapy. *Family Networker*, 51–55.

6. Teenage Pregnancy and the Puerto Rican Family

Manuel J. Gutierrez, PhD
Research Director
ASPIRA Inc. of Pennsylvania
Philadelphia, Pennsylvania

R ecent census data indicate that there is a wide discrepancy between Spanish-origin families and non-Spanish origin families in the rates of female-headed families in the United States. For the population at large, 15.7% of all families are headed by a female with no husband present, whereas for Hispanics, 23% of all families are single parent, female-headed families (U.S. Bureau of the Census, 1985). A closer look at specific Hispanic subgroups reveals that there are even more pronounced differences among the subgroups: for Mexicans, the rate of female-headed households is 18.6%, for Puerto Ricans 44%, for Cubans 16%, for Central or South Americans 21.9%, and for other Spanish-origins 21.3%. Thus, the prevalence of female-headed Puerto Rican families living on the mainland is at least twice as high as that in any other Hispanic group living in the United States (U.S. Bureau of the Census, 1985). In general, Puerto Ricans also exhibit a higher rate of having never married than other Hispanic subgroups. Furthermore, the divorce rate for Puerto Ricans (8.2%) is only second to that of the Cubans (8.4%), but much higher than that of Mexicans (5.4%). In addition, of all the Hispanic subgroups, Puerto Ricans have the highest rate (42%) of families below the poverty level (U.S. Bureau of the Census, 1985), which is highly correlated with the lack of a male wage earner in the household.

Note: The author wishes to thank Braulio Montalvo and Nell Anderson for their valuable comments and suggestions.

Little is presently known about the causes for these disparities among Hispanic subgroups. While all subgroups share the same language and Spain's cultural heritage, there are historical and migratory differences which appear to contribute to observed disparities. More cross-cultural research among Hispanic subgroups is urgently needed to clarify familial and cultural similarities and differences after controlling for socioeconomic status.

Darabi and Ortiz (1987) have provided a partial explanation to the above-noted disparity in rates of female-headed families with no husband present. In a secondary analysis of the National Longitudinal Survey of Labor Market Experience, they found that most first births occur within marriage for young women of Mexican origin, while most first births to Puerto Rican young women are premarital. This difference cannot be ascribed to age at marriage, since both Mexicans and Puerto Ricans marry at approximately the same age. In order to explain this difference, the authors point to the strong norms proscribing premarital sexual activity among Mexicans.

Because the birth statistics for Puerto Ricans are closer to those of Blacks than to those of Mexicans or Whites, Darabi (1986) has suggested that the northeast urban areas where most Puerto Ricans (and many Blacks) live may have an environmental impact on Puerto Rican families. The number of premarital births is inversely related to socioeconomic status for Puerto Ricans; higher status is related to fewer premarital births (Darabi & Ortiz, 1987). The fact that 42% of all Puerto Rican families live in poverty engenders a poverty cycle; young teenagers in low-income, female-headed, families become pregnant and themselves become family heads. The effects of recency of migration to the U.S. and other family and educational characteristics are important factors that need to be examined in cross-cultural research.

HISTORICAL CONTEXT

Historically, female teenage marriages and teenage births were common in Puerto Rico, as in most Third World, underdeveloped, agrarian countries. Large families were needed to share in the demanding agricultural tasks necessary for survival. The industrialization of Puerto Rico in the 1950s brought one of the largest migrations to the U.S. mainland. This was a product of a deliberate government policy, as the island needed an escape valve in order to deal with its overpopulation and lack of jobs. Since then, the Puerto Rican migration, primarily a rural migration, has been a continuing process that reflects the economic upheavals on the mainland as well as on the island. It has been undeterred by immigration quotas because Puerto Ricans born on the island were granted U.S. citizenship in 1917. Currently, there are 2.5 million Puerto Ricans who reside in the United States, while 3.5 million live in Puerto Rico.

Garcia-Coll's studies (in press) on teenage childbearing in Puerto Rico suggest that within an urban, low socioeconomic status population, early marriage and childbearing appear to be accepted as part of normal adolescent growth and development. While her samples were very small, she found that families in Puerto Rico commonly accept an unexpected teenage pregnancy as long as a marriage occurs. Thus, there seem to be differences between the Puerto Rican experience on the island and that on the mainland. It is possible that the socioeconomic and familial characteristics of those who choose to migrate to the mainland are different. After all, these families are facing impoverished resources and seek to improve their lot in the United States. Also contributing to the mainland experience are the stresses caused by deplorable living conditions in urban ghettos as well as by the demands exerted by an unfamiliar culture and a strange language. It may be that these forces manifest themselves in a powerful manner so that the traditional values of the Puerto Rican family are challenged and often replaced by predominant values of low socioeconomic status urban ghetto dwellers.

However, there is evidence to suggest that many families do manage to preserve traditional values in spite of the social and economic pressures that they face on a day-to-day basis. For example, in a recent longitudinal study of Puerto Rican young adults in Philadelphia with a mean age of 21.5 years, 26% of the 172 women surveyed reported that they had not yet had intercourse, and another 16% reported that they first had intercourse after marriage (Gutierrez, Montalvo, Armstrong, Webb, & Pickens, 1987). These findings support the notion that traditional family values (e.g., virginity and marriage) are still prevalent in a significant segment of this population.

When examining the teenage pregnancy phenomenon among Puerto Ricans, it is essential to consider contraceptive practices within a historical context. Surprisingly, by 1965 Puerto Rico had become the country with the highest per capita rate of sterilizations in the world (Ramirez de Arellano & Seipp, 1983). This was the result of a government-sponsored campaign in the 1950s and 1960s that promoted sterilization as the safest and most practical means of birth control. A thorough and chilling exposé of this campaign, including its misinformation efforts (e.g., women were told that the operation could be reversed whenever they wanted), is presented in the award-winning documentary "La Operación" by Ana Maria Garcia (1982). Sterilization, then, has been the recommended and accepted means of controlling their fertility for at least two generations of Puerto Rican women.

Another historical factor involves the field testing of birth control pills in Puerto Rico in the 1950s. These tests resulted in serious detrimental effects for many women, as the dosage was much higher during the field tests than it was later when the pills were marketed in the United States and Europe. Thus, Puerto Rican women have been fearful of using birth control pills, even though the dosage was subsequently reduced. Consequently, a fairly common practice among many Puerto Rican women has been to not use birth control pills regularly, and to rely on sterilization to limit the number of children. Religious beliefs and idealization of large families also play a role in the low levels of contraceptive practices among Puerto Ricans.

FAMILY IDEOLOGY

A series of focus group sessions held separately with pregnant Puerto Rican teenagers and their mothers helped in clarifying family processes and family ideology in matters of sex and adolescent pregnancy (Rivera, Gutierrez & Montalvo, 1987). None of the fifteen teenagers, all in junior high school, reported using contraceptives prior to their pregnancies. Furthermore, while the reasons for not using birth control were varied (e.g., "didn't think I would get pregnant," "was embarrassed to get it," "wanted it 'natural'"), most of the girls did not plan to use birth control in the future. When asked what method they would choose if they wanted to avoid more children, *all* of the 15 girls chose sterilization ("tying the tubes"). The cultural legacy is inescapable.

All the girls reported that they had kept their sexual activity a secret from their mothers and that their mothers, who were the first to know in the family, had generally become very upset at the news of the pregnancy. All sorts of recriminations and explosive confrontations had occurred; some parents insisted that the pregnant teenager move in with her boyfriend and his parents as they claimed that she had become the responsibility of the boy and his parents. The reactions of the girls' fathers were predictable: they became enraged and depressed at the loss of their daughters' innocence. At this point, the mothers played a crucial "bridging" role, shifting their attention from their daughters to their husbands in order to calm and help them recover from their feelings of dejection. In some cases, the mother, while still giving her daughter the "cold shoulder" treatment in order to make her feel guilty, simultaneously began transacting with her husband in order to seek a practical solution to the situation. In other cases, the father has been the one who strived to accept the situation and find a practical solution while the mother sulked and rejected her daughter. In a few cases, the parents received the pregnancy as a "blessed" event from the beginning and made few recriminations.

When examining family ideology, it is important to consider several factors. First, familial acceptance of a premarital teenage pregnancy seems to be strongly determined by the family's expectations of fulfillment by the birth of a baby. While this is a common expectation of the teenagers, in the case of Puerto Rican families it tends to also be a strong expectation of the *teenagers' mothers*. For many of these mothers, sterilization or other factors (e.g., separation or divorce) may have ended their reproductive years. Thus, the birth of a new baby is viewed as a reaffirmation of their own motherhood, even though their daughters are the ones who are giving birth. In addition, Puerto Rican families regard babies as generating happiness and pride, notwithstanding the economic and social consequences of child-rearing. As a popular saying indicates, *Donde comen muchos come otro* (Where many eat, another can eat, too). Finally, there is a strong antiabortion sentiment among Puerto Rican families; this reflects both religious beliefs and cultural considerations. Even when young mothers are unable to take care of their babies, they usually have relatives or close friends willing to assume responsibility for the child. Thus, it is very common to find families with *hijos de crianza* (unofficial foster children). These ideological considerations are presented as generalizations as there are always exceptions to the rule.

A THERAPEUTIC MODEL

In general, it is possible to identify five stages in the family's reaction to a teenage pregnancy. These stages are natural family processes likely to occur in a majority of low socioeconomic status families. Recency of migration, degree of religiosity, parental education, and other family based variables may affect the intensity, duration, and fixation of each stage, as well as the final resolution of the situation. For each of the stages described below, there are some specific suggestions offered for the therapist:

1. **Initial parental rejection.** This is likely to occur in one-parent as well as in two-parent families; it is a predictable reaction based on traditional cultural patterns. At this stage, the therapist should respond to the parental indignation with understanding and respect. The girl's situation should not be emphasized. The therapist should be perceived by the parents as someone who appreciates the magnitude of their disappointment and hurt, and as someone who can be trusted. This stage is usually brief.

2. **Intense turmoil.** The news of a teenage pregnancy typically leads to strong emotional outbursts and postures in family members; threats of murder and suicide are not uncommon, though these are seldom carried out. The pregnant girl may move with her boyfriend and his parents or may run away during this intense period when issues of family honor and responsibility predominate. This is a very difficult period for the family and for the therapist. The therapist needs to become more active and take charge during this stage. Crisis management techniques and involving available familial and community resources are required. The therapist needs to restrain impulses, maintain safeguards, and normalize the situation. Physical distance between the pregnant girl and her parents may be needed, in order to maintain appropriate bound-

aries. Attempts to preserve some communication, through third parties if necessary, should be stressed. The duration of this stage ranges from a few days to several weeks. The therapist should be alert for signs indicative of the next stage.

3. Efforts at accommodation. In this stage, one parent (usually the mother) or another close relative moves to seek acceptance of the pregnant teenager from the parent who is most distressed (usually the father). There may be a certain ritual or protocol in which the peacemaker and then the pregnant teenager ask forgiveness from that parent. Preliminary familial support is subsequently extended to the pregnant girl. This is a very important stage, where the therapist works to allow the offended parent to save face and appeals to his or her religious and/or family values for forgiveness and acceptance.

4. Practical solution. After some accommodation and acceptance have been attained, the family is ready to deal realistically with the situation and reach a practical solution. The family already accepts the inevitability of the situation and adjusts to it in some fashion; they are ready to deal with the issues of marriage, living arrangements, financial support, continued schooling, etc. At this stage, the therapist needs to be task-oriented and practical. By now, more emphasis needs to be given to the girl's situation and to her wishes. The therapist needs to help both parents and daughter develop realistic expectations.

5. Post-birth accommodation. The arrival of the baby poses a new challenge to the family and assigns new roles to each family member. Issues of child care responsibilites and child rearing practices emerge during this period. Attitudes may soften some more with the arrival of the baby, as the teenager is perceived more as a woman and less as a youngster. The birth of the baby should be used by the therapist to reflect back on the initial crisis and to emphasize the family's accomplishments in handling it. The family should face new tasks with a sense of competence, not with feelings of failure and dejection.

CASE EXAMPLES

The following case examples illustrate the stages that typically occur when Puerto Rican families are faced with a pregnant teenager. While these stages represent natural processes, therapeutic interventions are often needed in order to defuse emotions, facilitate successful transitions and guide the family toward enhanced functioning. The author was the therapist in both cases presented below.

Elena: The Case of the Girl Who Could Not "Marry in White"

Elena, a 16 year old girl, was the youngest of two siblings in an intact Puerto Rican family that had migrated to the U.S. in the 1960s. Both parents worked, and the family could be described as a lower middle class family. When Elena became pregnant she decided to tell her mother first, but was not able to tell her face-to-face. Instead, she wrote her a letter and left it on her mother's night table.

In this letter, Elena explained shamefully that she had become pregnant and explained why she had become sexually active with her boyfriend. Elena wrote that she had lost her virginity 3 years earlier when her maternal uncle had seduced her. She had been unable to confide in her mother or anyone else at the time, as she felt extremely ashamed and thought that the consequences of her telling would be much greater than the consequences of secrecy. In her mind, she had disgraced herself by losing her virginity and could never "marry in white," since she would not be a virgin bride. She acceded to her 18-year-old boyfriend's demands for sex because she felt that she had nothing to safeguard for the future. In her mind, a traditional wedding was never to be.

While she did not fully articulate the alternatives, she proceeded to move toward one: getting pregnant and then marrying her boyfriend. While pregnancy was not the immediate desired outcome, it was not an outcome to avoid either. As in a majority of cases, the couple did not use any birth control method. The explicit agreement was that they would marry if Elena became pregnant and, indeed, they planned to do so when the pregnancy was confirmed. However, the boyfriend had no job and his family did not offer to support the young couple and their baby.

Elena's parents were extremely upset when they learned of the pregnancy. Her father was devastated, and her mother was critical and rejecting. Furthermore, they decided that Elena had dishonored the family and would have to leave home. Fortunately, an aunt took Elena in and acted as the all-important "bridge" between her and her parents. It was at that time that Elena was referred for therapy.

While Elena's parents gave permission for her to become involved in therapy, they refused to participate themselves. The therapist worked with the parents sending messages through a caseworker who knew Elena's family well. The messages were simple and emphasized the therapist's concern for Elena's well-being and her need for family support. Although efforts to involve the parents more directly in therapy were unsuccessful, Elena's father began to move toward acceptance of the situation. Working individually with Elena, the therapist encouraged her to continue communicating with her parents (often through her aunt or through the caseworker), and not to become discouraged by their initial reaction.

Elena and her father were reconciled after he had vented his anger and disappointment. However, the same was not true for her mother, who continued to be critical of Elena and failed to accept that her own brother had sexually abused her daughter. Meanwhile, Elena continued in school, determined to finish her education. After a few months, Elena's parents allowed her to move back home. In a final show of hostility and rejection, Elena's mother went to Puerto Rico to visit her family when Elena was due to give birth.

After the birth of the baby, Elena's mother could no longer maintain her rejecting posture. Upon her return from Puerto Rico, she brought greetings from the extended family as well as an assortment of baby presents and hand-made baby clothes. The entire family was now ready for re-engagement and accommodation. New issues emerged (e.g., Elena's continuing relationship with her boyfriend and child care), but this time the family dealt with these issues within a context of acceptance of the reality and a willingness to assume new roles. Therapy focused on helping Elena sort out her feelings, supporting her as she attempted to reconcile with her parents and plan for her future. Some sessions with Elena included her boyfriend who had decided to join the Army in order to escape the conflicts with Elena's parents and as a source of self-development. Initially, he maintained contact with Elena and planned to marry her, but eventually lost interest in her and married someone else. Elena continued to live with her parents while she finished high school and subsequently got a job.

Five years later, Elena is a single-parent head of a household. She holds a good-paying secretarial position, which allows her to rent her own apartment. Her mother, who took care of her son before he attended school, now takes care of him after school until Elena picks him up after work; her mother also babysits when Elena goes out on weekends. Elena feels that she and her son have a good future.

Lucy: The Case of the "Rotten Apple"

Lucy, a 15 year old girl, was the oldest of six children in an intact Puerto Rican family. There were five sisters and one brother; the boy was the youngest child. Lucy's parents had migrated to the mainland soon after their marriage. Her father was employed, and the family was a lower middle class family. In addition to his full-time work, Lucy's father was also a leader of a Catholic sodality group. The parents were very strict, forbidding the girls to go out with boys or even to attend parties outside their church. Social activities for the family were restricted to church activities and some family events. Lucy's father complained that he did not even like to spend a great deal of time with his extended family because they would frequently argue. Against this very strict background in which the parents expected virginity, an approved courtship, and a church wedding for all the daughters, Lucy became pregnant by her first, secret, boyfriend. She had not used birth control, because she did not think she would get pregnant. The boy was not much older than Lucy; he had already dropped out of school and had been in trouble with the law. Furthermore, he had already impregnated another girl. Abortion was out of the question both for Lucy's parents and for Lucy herself. She loved this boy and wanted to have his baby. Furthermore, her world was crumbling; she was ostracized by her own family and many of her friends, and her education was in jeopardy. She perceived having a child as the only tangible reward she could obtain from that situation, given the fact that her parents would not allow her to leave home and live with her boyfriend.

When first seen in therapy, Lucy's father presented a rigid posture of offended pride and honor. He had declared Lucy a "rotten apple" and was primarily concerned about the negative role model that she provided for her younger sisters. He wanted to send her to Puerto Rico to live with relatives in order to keep her away from her sisters and to keep her away from him; he stated that he felt only shame and disgust when he looked at her. Lucy's mother was very depressed and ineffectual; she was unable to deal with her husband's anger or to provide any support for Lucy. She deferred all decisions to her husband.

When the family sought therapy, mainly because of a social worker's insistence, the family was in the middle of the turmoil stage. There were few indications that they would be able to reach any accommodation. Sending Lucy to Puerto Rico was not perceived as an effort at accommodation but rather as a punishment and a banishment from the family. The therapist attempted several maneuvers to deal with the father's extreme rigidity and the mother's ineffectiveness. However, efforts to strengthen the mother's position failed because she would always return to a submissive position. Lucy's rebelliousness and determination contrasted sharply with her mother's extreme submissiveness. It seemed that Lucy had been destined in her family to challenge her father's patriarchal and authoritarian role. As the challenger, however, she was paying a hefty price for her actions. Efforts to help Lucy communicate directly with her father were only partially successful, because they were too angry with each other. Although Lucy presented an "I don't care" attitude on the outside, she cared very much about her father's total rejection of her.

A breakthrough was made when the therapist decided to spend time alone with Lucy's father in each of the family sessions. This allowed the therapist to talk to Lucy's father man-to-man and father-to-father in a context where he would not lose face in front of his family. These sessions allowed for an exploration of the father's hurt and disappointment, which were the basis for his anger and rigid posture. He appeared to enjoy engaging the therapist in a discussion of religion, which he used to justify his behavior. When Lucy's father emphasized the morality of the Old Testament, the therapist refocused the discussion on themes of forgiveness and acceptance from the New Testament.

Soon after these discussions with Lucy's father began, her mother started to show more external support for Lucy by taking her to buy maternity clothes and even accompanying her to the doctor. It appeared that, as her father softened in his attitude toward Lucy, her mother saw the opportunity to move closer to her, knowing that she would not offend her husband by doing so. Of course, Lucy's father never openly admitted that he was becoming more accepting of the situation, but he stopped talking about sending Lucy to Puerto Rico and stopped calling her a "rotten apple." While not totally accepting the situation, this was as close as Lucy's father would get to a practical solution. He allowed his wife to continue doing things for Lucy, but he never abandoned his basic posture toward Lucy; he continued to be aloof and uncommunicative with her.

The birth of the baby produced no significant changes in the family's functioning. Lucy's mother willingly shared in child care responsibilities, knowing that her husband would not oppose this. Lucy was responsible toward her baby, but decided to drop out of school. The family discontinued therapy after the birth of the baby.

Follow-up, two years later, revealed that Lucy had maintained her relationship with her boyfriend and had given birth to a second baby. She was still living at home and had not returned to school. Her boyfriend continued to have trouble with the law and was not committed to living with her or to supporting the children. The family dynamics evidenced minimal change, except that both parents had assumed an attitude of resigned acceptance. For Lucy, her role as a mother was very important, but she seemed stuck in an unsupportive and destructive relationship with her boyfriend. The notion of attending a GED (General Equivalency Diploma) program to complete her high school education appeared to be more of a possibility at follow-up, although she still had not acted on the idea. The struggle continues for Lucy.

IMPLICATIONS

Historical and cultural determinants are important considerations when working with Puerto Rican families with pregnant teenagers. In spite of acculturation pressures, cultural legacies and traditional values still retain powerful influences on the Puerto Rican family on the mainland. A teenage pregnancy is a major crisis, usually resulting in extreme reactions, both negative and positive, within the family. A systems perspective is very helpful to the therapist because even during the most volatile periods, family members often tend to act in highly stereotypical ways. A therapist's understanding of the natural family processes that occur with the event of a teenager's pregnancy facilitates therapeutic interventions.

The observations presented in this chapter are meant as sources for hypotheses and as potential intervention pathways for the clinician engaging a Puerto Rican family with a pregnant teenager. They should not be taken as "cookbook recipes" that apply to all cases presenting the same dilemma. Nor are they to be taken as a substitute for a sound understanding of families regardless of their ethnic background. As Montalvo and Gutierrez (1983) have stated, the clini-

84   CLINICAL ISSUES IN SINGLE-PARENT HOUSEHOLDS

cian must guard against being swallowed by a family's cultural masks. While cultural patterns can sometimes enlighten certain family dilemmas, they can also obscure maladaptive patterns within the family and fool the clinician.

In a broader context, it is critical to develop policies that increase the range of life options for both male and female Puerto Rican teenagers. At present, Puerto Ricans have one of the highest dropout rates for any ethnic group in the United States, a situation that prevents a significant number of Puerto Rican youngsters from planning or even considering other career options. Many girls perceive early motherhood as one of the few viable and acceptable career options. Clearly, there must be major interventions and initiatives within urban educational systems in order to arrest the school dropout epidemic among Puerto Rican youths. Their futures and their children's futures are at stake!

REFERENCES

Darabi, K. (1986). *Teenage pregnancy and childbearing among Hispanic women.* Paper presented at the Coalition of Hispanic Health and Human Services Organization National Conference, New York.

Darabi, K., & Ortiz, V. (1987). Childbearing among young Latino women in the United States. *American Journal of Public Health, 77*, 25–28.

Garcia, A.M. (1982). *La operación* [Documentary film]. New York: Tricontinental Films.

Garcia-Coll, C. (in press). The consequences of teenage childbearing in traditional Puerto Rican culture. In L. Nugent, B.M. Lester, & T. Brazelton (Eds.), *Cultural context of infancy.* Princeton, NJ: Ablex.

Gutierrez, M., Montalvo, B., Armstrong, K., Webb, D., & Pickens, G. (1987). *Premarital sexual relations and pregnancy among Puerto Rican youths.* Final report submitted to the Office of Adolescent Pregnancy Programs, U.S. Department of Health and Human Services.

Montalvo, B., & Gutierrez, M. (1983). A perspective for the use of the cultural dimension in family therapy. In C.J. Falicov (Ed.), *Cultural perspectives in family therapy.* Rockville, MD: Aspen Publishers, Inc.

Ramirez de Arellano, A., & Seipp, C. (1983). *Colonialism, Catholicism, and contraception: A history of birth control in Puerto Rico.* Chapel Hill, NC: University of North Carolina Press.

Rivera, L., Gutierrez, M., & Montalvo, B. (1987). *From hope to despair: Teenage pregnancy among Puerto Ricans.* Unpublished manuscript.

U.S. Bureau of the Census. (1985). *Persons of Spanish origin in the United States* (Current Population Reports, Series P-20, No. 403). Washington, DC.

7. Coping with the Young Handicapped Child in the Single-Parent Family: An Ecosystemic Perspective

C. Wayne Jones, PhD
Staff Psychologist
Preschool Services
Philadelphia Child Guidance Clinic
Philadelphia, Pennsylvania

U nfortunately, there is some evidence that single-parent households have a disproportionate number of handicapped children (Bristol, Reichle, & Thomas, 1986). This may be due to a higher rate of marital dissolution among families that have a handicapped child (Bristol, Schopler, & McConnaughey, 1984) or to the higher percentage of retarded children born to low-income, never-married mothers (Broman, Nichols, & Kennedy, 1975). The numerous additional physical and affective demands that accompany most handicapping conditions often further tax the single-parent family's already strained resources. It is hardly surprising, therefore, that single mothers with a young handicapped child report feeling more stressed than do married mothers with such a child (Beckman-Bell, 1981; Holroyd, 1974). There is a paucity of literature, however, that examines issues unique to single mothers with a young handicapped child.

Relevant clinical issues stem from three different domains within the single parent's ecosystem: (1) the individual child, (2) the family and personal network, and (3) the professional network. Within an ecosystemic framework, it is assumed that coping outcomes are a function of the "goodness of fit" between demands and resources across these three highly interrelated domains within the ecosystem (Aponte, 1976; Keeney, 1983).

Note: The author would like to express his appreciation to Chris Maisto, PhD for her constructive comments on earlier versions of this manuscript.

Of course, single-parent families are not a homogeneous group. They differ in their socioeconomic status, ethnicity, developmental status within the individual and family life cycles, the cause of the single parenthood (e.g., death of a spouse, desertion, separation or divorce, or out-of-wedlock birth), and the head of the family (i.e., father or mother). While the nature of the demands associated with the care of a handicapped child is similar for all these sub-groups, the most stressed subsample of single-parent families probably consists of the low-income or working-class, never-married, mother-headed families that have a handicapped infant or preschooler.

HANDICAP-RELATED REALITY STRESSORS

Certain child care tasks and emotional demands are thrust on the family of a handicapped child just by the fact of the handicap. Wolfensberger (1967) termed these demands "reality stressors." The severity of the handicapping condition and the degree of certainty regarding the diagnosis of the condition, its causes, and its prognosis partially determine the nature of these reality stressors. In addition, they affect parents' confidence in their ability to deal with the handicap and the continuation of parents' connections within their social networks.

Handicap Severity

Generally, the more severely disabling the handicap, the more stressed the parent (Beckman, 1983; Tew & Laurence, 1975). Three aspects of a handicap seem to determine its effect on family members: (1) the degree to which the handicapped child can assist in his or her own care, (2) the child's level of social responsiveness, and (3) the number and magnitude of unusual behaviors that the child exhibits.

Among the severely disabling conditions are physical impairments (e.g., cerebral palsy, spina bifida, or muscular dystrophy), particularly when they leave the child nonambulatory. Children with such conditions require considerable assistance with basic self-help skills, such as feeding, dressing, carrying, toileting, and exercising in special ways. For those physically impaired children who are also retarded or incapable of speech, the parent must be hypervigilant to determine what the child needs. Parental fears of infections, bed sores, and falls are realistic for many of these children. Furthermore, many physically impaired children require periodic surgical procedures, requiring parents to spend considerable time in medical clinics and hospitals.

The care of a physically impaired child causes family stress in many ways. For the low-income single parent, the cost of special equipment and transportation for medical care often becomes a very stressful issue. The parent who must handle all the extra tasks, in addition to raising other children, may have insufficient time or energy left to participate in activities with other adults or to maintain ongoing relationships with adult friends; yet these activities and relationships can facilitate parental adjustment (Jones, 1986).

Children who are autistic or have pervasive developmental disorders often require the same extensive care that physically impaired children require, but these children show little or no positive affective responsiveness to the parent who provides this care. In addition, these children often show numerous bizarre behaviors, such as tantrums and stereotypical, self-stimulatory rituals. At times, they may even injure themselves, seemingly impervious to the pain. It is not surprising that, of all the families with a handicapped child, families with an autistic child report the greatest amount of stress (Holroyd & McArthur, 1976).

Children who are socially responsive, despite severe physical handicaps, quickly develop likeable attributes and traits that facilitate bonding; they are able to give something back to the parents who give them care. When interacting with these children, parents do not relate to them as generic "handicapped children." Autistic children, on the other hand, give little or nothing back to their parents, which makes it extraordinarily difficult for their parents to remain affectively bonded to them and continue to give them all the extra time and energy that they need. A parent who must struggle repeatedly through feeding a tactilely defensive child who makes no eye contact and spits the food out as fast as it is given to him is likely to perceive the mealtime ritual very differently from the way that the parent whose child smiles warmly and coos during feeding perceives it. When the parent begins to show frustration and to establish an emotional distance from the child, outsiders may add insult to injury by hinting that the child's problem may be due to an unloving parent.

Because of the huge number of additional child care tasks associated with both physical impairments and autism, parents of children with these handicaps cannot on a whim run to the store, visit a neighbor, or see a movie. For the parent of an autistic child, unusual behaviors such as hand flapping, stereotypical rocking, echolalia, and severe tantrums can make any public venture not only embarrassing, but also physically taxing. It is little wonder that these families often elect to stay home, thereby risking the loosening of some ties with peers (Farber, 1968; Kazak & Marvin, 1984).

The prospect of a child's lifelong dependence can be overwhelming for a parent, particularly for a younger never-married woman who had planned to enroll in school or develop a career when the child was older. Parents of severely handicapped children are also likely to feel sadness and grief evoked by the loss of the anticipated normal child (Moses, 1983), as well as anger and embarrassment evoked by the social stigma that often accompanies certain handicaps (Goffman, 1963). Because parents may be struggling with all these emotions at the same time that they are toiling with the extra day-to-day basic child care tasks, they often appear very fatigued. This is not to be confused with clinical depression, however.

When a child's handicap is severe enough to be noticed in any family, the meaning attributed to the handicap and the emotions that follow in low-income single-parent families are probably not very different from those in more middle-class intact families. There may be a difference between the reactions of these two groups, however, when the handicap is more specific, is less visible, and requires less additional care (e.g., mild-to-moderate developmental delays that are not accompanied by significant motor problems). Low-income, less educated, single-parent families are less likely to identify these handicaps as serious stressors. In fact, these handicaps may go unnoticed in a low-income single-parent family until a pediatrician or early childhood educator brings a problem such as an articulation difficulty or limited expressive speech to the family's attention. The most recognizable stress for such a family is that introduced by teachers, speech and language therapists, and other helping professionals who may perceive the problem as more serious than the family perceives it.

Ambiguity in Diagnosis

Some severely handicapping conditions, such as autism and pervasive developmental disorders, are initially subtle and, thus, may not be officially diagnosed until the child is 2 or 3 years old. Any ambiguity in the diagnosis of a child's handicap can create severe emotional strain for parents. Without an official diagnosis, parents have no clear way to determine whether the child's difficulties stem from the child's biological make-up or from their misguided parenting efforts. Until they have a definite diagnosis, parents do not know what they can realistically expect of the child or of themselves, which may fuel any preexisting conflict among family members about parenting issues.

The diagnosis of autism is particularly ambiguous, as the autistic child may appear physically normal. In order to resolve this very stressful state of ambiguity, parents are likely either to deny and minimize the child's differences or to blame themselves for failing to be effective parents. Professionals may unknowingly reinforce the denial or misplaced feelings of guilt by responding to parental concerns with brief, vague explanations.

Early uncertainty and ambiguity about the nature and cause of an autistic child's handicap not only may foster disagreements between parents and professionals and between parents and other family members, but also may increase conflict or emotional distance between parents and their peers. A mother whose son has obvious physical deformities is more likely to receive sympathy from her friends when he throws his food across the room during a tantrum than is the mother of a child whose handicaps are not so visible. The latter mother, as Bristol (1984) noted, is more likely to encounter only hostility and unsolicited advice on child-rearing, further heightening her sense of embarrassment and shame.

Clinical Implications of Reality Stressors

A therapist who is working with a family that has a handicapped child should first learn about the specific day-to-day care that the child requires because of the handicap and the degree of professional certainty about the diagnosis and causes of the condition. This information helps the clinician (1) to determine which aspects of the family's problems may be directly attributable to the demands imposed by the handicap and which originate in more basic family structure problems, and (2) to join with the family (Harris, 1984). The degree to which the family understands the diagnosis, its causes, and its prognosis is also critical. Very few handicapping conditions have clearly identifiable causes, and the family is likely to be struggling to accept this fact. The clinician can help by referring the family to professionals who can explain the medical or psychological test findings clearly and patiently. In the next section, factors within the family and personal network system will be examined in order to gain a better idea why some single-parents perceive the situation as more manageable than others, despite the reality stressors associated with the handicapping condition.

THE FAMILY AND PERSONAL NETWORK SYSTEM

Each family has its own idiosyncratic emotional issues and preferred style for handling routine functions. The reality stressors that accompany the presence of a handicapped child in the family, therefore, highlight different sensitive family emotional and structural issues in different families. It would be a serious error, therefore, for the therapist to treat such a family as though it were a generic "family of a handicapped child."

It would also be a serious error to treat the single-parent family generically. It is often assumed—incorrectly—that fathers are not involved in single-mother families and that the single mother does all the child-rearing alone. As Bristol (in press) noted, however, father involvement is a continuum in both single-parent and two-parent families. In traditional two-parent families, for example, it is not uncommon for mothers to perform most of the child care tasks with little assistance from fathers, even when the child is handicapped (Gallagher, Scharfman, & Bristol, 1984). Bristol (in press) found that single mothers named absent fathers as regular participants in approximately 20% of child care tasks; they named fathers as important sources of child care assistance five times as often as they named boyfriends.

In addition to fathers and boyfriends, single mothers often seek help from other family members and friends, such as an older sibling, the mother's mother, and father's mother, more distant relatives, or neighbors. A single parent is less likely to be parenting the child alone than is suggested by the term *single parent*. In fact, those single parents who have not been able to enlist the assistance of others in child care tasks are likely to be those adjusting most poorly (Beavers, Hampson, Hulgus, & Beavers, 1986).

Structural issues involving the parental subsystem are the most common problems for single parents who are raising a handicapped child. These parents may find it difficult to form a workable parental coalition with other family members, or they may become over- or underinvolved with the handicapped child. The way in which family members deal with these structural issues reflects their ability to enter into conflict and resolve it effectively (Minuchin, Rosman, & Baker, 1978). Given the ambiguities often associated with raising a handicapped child, this ability can be a pivotal factor in the family's adjustment to this challenge.

The Parental Coalition

A strong parental coalition, such as that between the mother and her own mother, is a feature of higher functioning single-parent families (Beavers et al., 1986; Minuchin, Rosman, & Baker, 1978). In a successful coalition, all members of the parental subsystem feel capable and valued in their parenting efforts.

The single mother who feels that she alone understands the handicapped child's special needs may overfunction, thus underutilizing the helping efforts of other potential care-givers. On the other hand, the single mother who allows another care-giver to assume the primary responsibility for the child may feel increasingly incompetent and withdraw from participation in child-related decisions. The latter dysfunctional pattern occurs most frequently when the single mother remains in her own mother's home after the birth of the child, particularly if the single mother is older and is beginning to individuate. In one study of low-income, black single mothers who had a handicapped child and who were aged 24 and over, for example, those who were living in their parents' homes showed significantly greater personal distress than did those who were living independently (Jones, 1986). It appears that it is easier for the single mother to negotiate power issues around child care responsibilities with her own mother when there is some physical distance between them.

For younger single mothers, close proximity to their primary sources of support can be very functional. If her mother provides a major portion of the child care, the young mother is free to finish her education, get a job, and build good connections with peers. This very functional structural arrangement can become dysfunctional when the relationship system does not accommodate changes in the developmental needs of each of the family members, however.

Janice became pregnant at age 16. Because she was embarrassed and frightened by the pregnancy, she tried to keep it a secret; therefore, she received no prenatal care. Wendy was born 3 months premature with numerous medical complications that required around-the-clock monitoring after she left the hospital at 2 months of age. Janice's mother took full responsibility for the child initially, occasionally turning to the older sister of the baby's father for help. The father himself was never directly involved with either Wendy or Janice after the child's birth. While her mother overfunctioned as parent to her baby, Janice became peripheral to the parenting process. She completed high school and enrolled in a brief secretarial course at a community college.

This arrangement worked well for the family until Janice's mother, who had had few adult friends of her own at the time of Wendy's birth, began developing outside interests. This coincided with a decrease in the number of special child care demands posed by Wendy, as her condition was improving. However, because Janice had spent so little time with Wendy and knew little about how to take care of Wendy's special needs, she was frightened and angry when her mother began demanding that she take more responsibility for Wendy's care. The family sought therapy following a referral from Wendy's early intervention teacher, who described the ordinarily bubbly 3-year-old youngster as increasingly quiet and withdrawn.

Because of her mother's history of depression and social isolation, Janice had come to associate overt conflict with danger. Therefore, she was unable to negotiate power issues directly with her mother. Janice's solution was to move out of her mother's home and triangulate others into the conflict. She arranged to have Wendy divide her time every week so that she stayed sometimes with Janice, sometimes with members of the father's family, and sometimes with Janice's mother. This disrupted Wendy's sleep and feeding schedules and interfered with her attendance at school, where she had developed strong attachments. Wendy, a child who had necessarily been the center of attention all her life, suddenly found herself pushed to the periphery of the family's concerns, and she felt lost.

When Wendy's medical needs were very clear, her mother and her grandmother had been able to form a workable, although noncollaborative, parental coalition. As often occurs in non-collaborative parental subsystems, Janice was unable to step in and assume the parental role when her mother began to distance herself from it. This left a parental void for Wendy.

The inability to resolve conflict within the parental subsystem can result in more direct triangulation of the handicapped child. For example, the element of ambiguity associated with handicapping conditions often makes it difficult to know whether the child's limitations should be gently accepted or whether the child should be pushed to do more. When the single parent cannot enter into dialogue or agree with a partner around such issues, parental anxiety may become overfocused on the child, resulting in expectations that are too low or too high.

Ann was a very energetic 26-year-old never-married single parent who had very high expectations for both herself and others. She sought therapy for her 4-year-old, moderately retarded son because he tended to ignore her when she set limits and to become very uncooperative when she tried to prepare him for school by teaching him the *ABC*s. Given his developmental level, her expectations for the child were very unrealistic, and the boy had become so belligerent in response to the impossible demands placed on him that his behavior was making learning even more difficult for him. There was no one within the parental subsystem who would challenge her, however.

The intensity of Ann's demands on her son seemed to be fueled primarily by the extremely low expectations that his father and her brother held for him; they took a "hands off" approach. Thus, the boy's mother and father were unable to work together and plan appropriate ways to help the child develop. The lack of accurate professional information on the child's capabilities made this type of dialogue between the parents even more difficult. The father had never been included in any psychological or medical feedback sessions regarding his son. Furthermore, both parents had misconceptions about the term *retardation* and what it indicated about them as parents.

Organization around the Child

Because of the number and intensity of the extra tasks generally required by a handicapped child and the stigma of certain handicaps, some families organize around the handicapped child and make the child the central focus in the family (Berger, 1984). This approach is maladaptive to the extent that it slights the needs of other family members or severs relationships with those outside the family.

> Carol, a never-married 36-year-old single parent, already had two children known to be learning-disabled when she was told that her youngest son, Steven, was both moderately retarded and autistic. In her view, this diagnosis confirmed that she had "bad" genes and dashed all hope of ever marrying. Because Carol was not well linked within her network of friends and tended to be somewhat distrustful, she became extremely overprotective of her youngest son. She refused to allow the father, her older children, or teachers in her son's school more than 10 minutes access to him; she talked about him incessantly.
>
> Carol's oldest son, who tended to be overly responsible in a parentified manner, quickly found himself even more on the periphery of the family's emotional life. His grades soon began plummeting, which provoked the call to the therapist.
>
> Shaken by the seriousness of the youngest son's condition, the father began to avoid Carol, who was increasingly irritable and depressed. There was a longstanding conflict between Carol and the children's father about parenting roles. For 5 years, he had been an alcoholic and relatively peripheral as a parent. In the previous 2 years, however, he had stopped drinking and was attempting to gain a more active position within the family. No one was talking directly about the enormous amount of pain members were experiencing under these circumstances.

The opposite problem, of course, is insufficient organization around the handicapped child. Those families that are unwilling or unable to devote the additional energy and time required to meeting the special needs of the handcapped child tend to be "multiproblem families" (Greenspan, 1986). Some single parents are forced to expend so much of their energy on maintaining some form of intact household that they have little time left to share with the children. In these situations, the handicapped child's special needs may be minimized, and parental involvement with the child may not be adequate for the child's proper physical and emotional development. When the personal networks of these single parents are small and dominated primarily by kin, the risk of neglect and abuse is high (Salzinger, Kaplan, & Artemyeff, 1983; Wahler, 1980). These families do not often seek therapy voluntarily.

Clinical Implications of the Family and Network System

In working with the single-parent family of a handicapped child, it is particularly important for the clinician to identify and involve all relevant members of the parental subsystem. These individuals are the sources of instrumental and emotional support that the parent needs to raise a handicapped child successfully (Jones, 1986). In addition, when one or more members of the family are intensely organized around the handicapped child, the clinician must be prepared to pace therapy very slowly. Fear is the predominant emotion within these systems, and families that have a handicapped child can be driven into even further protective isolation if this fear is not taken into account.

For those single parents who incorporate others into the parental role, conflicts usually revolve around (1) who is in charge of which parental functions and (2) what is expected of the handicapped child. As with any family in therapy for a child-related problem, a major therapeutic goal in these families is to facilitate the negotiation of such conflicts among members of the parental subsystem. The clinician must take care to normalize and support the changing developmental needs of all individuals, while keeping a clear focus on the parenting needs of the handicapped child. Failure to negotiate these conflicts adequately within the parental subsystem may result in over- or under-organization of the family around the handicapped child.

For those isolated single parents who are raising the child alone, the incorporation of others into some minimal level of support around child care functions is an essential long-term goal. It may be necessary for the child's teacher or the clinician to become a temporary part of the parental subsystem until the parent begins building stronger connections with others. In fact, because of the heightened dynamic tension between the needs of the handicapped child and the needs of the other family members, the participation of a special educator sometimes facilitates the clinical work. If a strong collaborative relationship between the therapist and the teacher can be developed, the tendency to focus excessively on either the family's needs or the child's needs may be held in check. The child's teacher played a major role in the therapy of all three clinical cases discussed earlier.

For example, Wendy's mother and grandmother could be brought together and involved in a therapy contract only within a school setting where the teacher used her knowledge of Wendy to highlight the child's continued needs. Ann's expectations for her son, as well as those of the boy's father, became more realistic following several sessions in which a special educator helped the parents select developmentally appropriate toys and learn to use these materials to engage their son in a more playful way, creating a more successful experience for both the child and his parents. Carol's confidence was gradually strengthened and her network broadened by referring her son to an early intervention program that would not rush her separation from her son in the classroom.

As is evident in the way the therapist chose to treat these families, there is a larger professional system that can be tapped to provide these families with therapeutic opportunities. This larger system, however, can also promote dysfunctional intrafamilial patterns.

FAMILY TRANSACTIONS WITH PROFESSIONALS

Families with a young handicapped child must deal with many more community professionals than do other families. They may have continuing contact not only with the pediatrician, but also with special educators, speech and language therapists, physical or occupational therapists, psychologists, and social workers. While it is clearly a blessing for the child and family to have so many experts available, it can also be the source of much additional stress (Turnbull & Turnbull, 1978). For low-income single parents, adding this army of experts to the already extensive list of social service professionals that may be involved with their family may further loosen their sense of personal control over their own lives.

In addition to the ordinary unpleasantness associated with keeping so many appointments and providing so many outsiders with so much personal information, much of the stress in family-professional transactions stems from the tendency of physicians and educators to focus on the needs of the handicapped child and overlook the special needs of other family members. Professionals who do not think of the child within the context of the family are unlikely to ask about the family's agenda for the child and, therefore, may recommend tasks that are beyond the family's scope of interest or ability, placing parents in a double bind (Foster, Berger, & McLean, 1981). When a parent does not follow these treatment prescriptions, the professionals may question the parent's commitment to the child. When the parent complies fully with the professionals' recommendations, the child may gain—but the rest of the family may suffer from neglect.

Early negative experiences with professionals may impair the family's ability to establish effective long-term working relationships with them. This can be particularly unfortunate for the family of a child whose handicap requires professional care for a lifetime. Two early points of family-professional contact that carry particularly strong implications for future transactions include the initial diagnostic sessions and the child's entry into an early intervention setting.

Diagnostic Feedback Sessions

As noted by Berger and Foster (1986), the time of diagnosis

> is a period in which family members are very concerned with understanding the ramifications of the child's handicap, with constructing an explanation of the origin of the handicapping condition, with interpreting the handicapping condition to other members of the social network, and with obtaining services for the child. (p. 256)

Therefore, families turn to professionals for clear and digestible information about the child at this time. Family members may be most emotionally vulnerable at the time of diagnosis, however, making some information particularly difficult to hear.

Professionals who are uncomfortable when they must deliver a diagnosis of a condition that has no cure may be overly brief and may clutter their explanations with jargon, leaving family members even more confused and anxious. As mentioned earlier, parents may fear that they have caused the child's handicap, and failure to address this emotion-laden question clearly may intensify their confusion. The less adjusted, guilt-ridden parent may incorrectly assume that the professional's discomfort is proof that worse information is being withheld. Such a parent may suffer in silence, becoming increasingly protective of the handicapped child. If the parent is particularly assertive and continues to question the impatient physician or psychologist about the findings, the desire for precise information may be misidentified as difficulty in dealing with the diagnosis, and the parent may be referred for therapy. For the parent who is denying the diagnosis, an uninformative diagnostic feedback session may reinforce the denial.

On the other hand, professionals may provide very clear information to family members, but these family members may angrily reject the diagnosis at first. If the professional aggressively pursues the issue, viewing this reaction as evidence of parental psychopathology rather than as a plea for time to digest very painful information, the parent may temporarily withdraw from professional networks. This prevents the parent's gradual and appropriate understanding of the handicap.

Professionals must carefully consider which family members should participate in the diagnostic feedback session and schedule the session accordingly. If the session is held at a time convenient for the professional (i.e., during the day), only the family members who are unemployed, regardless of their position vis-a-vis the child, may be able to attend; this may create additional problems. If only the grandmother can attend, for example, the natural mother, who may be struggling to take charge of her child, may be placed in a position subordinate to the grandmother, who now is more the expert than she. Similarly, if an absent father who participates in child care tasks cannot attend the session, he may become even more peripheral. These considerations apply not only to the initial diagnostic session, but also to all subsequent psychological, educational, and medical feedback sessions in which the child's progress is reviewed.

Involvement in Educational Interventions

Staff members in educational settings for young handicapped children generally have a strong interest in parent involvement. Parents typically become involved through classroom volunteer work, the development of individualized education programs (IEPs), and parent group meetings. Such involvement can communicate hope to parents, normalize their concerns about their child, improve their understanding of their child's strengths and needs, and broaden their repertoire of ways to work with the child at home. The strong staff orientation toward "intervention" that is partly responsible for these opportunities can also contribute to the maintenance of dysfunctional family situations, however.

For example, parents who feel overly responsible for the handicapping condition may have an exceptionally difficult time saying "no" to the numerous exercises, meetings, and evaluations that school staff recommend. If these guilt-ridden parents do all of the tasks that are prescribed, however, they become increasingly organized around the needs of the child, possibly neglecting their own needs and those of their other children. Before assigning tasks, staff members should ask parents to describe their daily schedules or describe who is available in their networks to assist them. Staff may misinterpret parents' anxiety as a request for more tasks; in reality, these parents may simply be searching for an expert who will tell them that they have done enough and can relax.

For the single mother whose self-esteem is already low as a result of criticism from her family of origin, failure to follow through on tasks recommended by the school staff may intensify her perception of herself as incompetent. If the next feedback session on her child's progress happens to show little gain, which is often the case with the more severe handicapping conditions—regardless of teacher and parent effort—this perception of incompetence is likely to be confirmed, both in the school and family context. In a sense, school staff unwittingly enter into a coalition with family members against this parent.

Single parents who maintain a low level of involvement with the school, preferring to work or to take advantage of a much needed respite and simply relax, risk being viewed by staff as "uninterested" in their children. Staff in educational settings sometimes mistake parental refusal to make the handicapped child the central focus of their lives as neglect. When this occurs, the child may be viewed as a victim and triangulated into conflict between the family and the school staff (Berger, 1984). A parent's rejection of the role of assistant to the expert and refusal to carry out an agenda that is not the family agenda can be a healthy response, however.

Clinical Implications of Family Transactions with Professionals

When a single-parent family with a handicapped child has been referred for therapy, the clinician should thoroughly assess the family's earlier relationships with professionals. The referral for therapy may be the result of a conflict with professionals who see the family as troubled or resistant because of the family's failure to follow through on the professionals' recommendations. On the other hand, the family may seek therapy voluntarily because family members believe that their failure to live up to the (unrealistic) expectations of those in their professional network must be their own fault. It is very important not to validate their status as "patients," but instead to normalize their dealings with any service agency with which they are in conflict.

Because it is likely that service agencies will be permanent fixtures in the lives of single parents with a handicapped child, clinicians should help these parents develop skills to obtain services that they need from professionals and to refuse services that they do not need. For example, IEP meetings are often intimidating to parents who do not understand the professional jargon employed by staff; therapists can empower parents by preparing them with questions and explaining the options generally open to them in school settings.

CONCLUSION

The expectations of a therapist who does not understand the day-to-day ramifications of the specific handicap on both the child and the parent may be out of step with the family's reality. Furthermore, the therapist will be unable to determine what kinds of concrete resources are required to improve family functioning. Wolfensberger (1967) noted that the parents of handicapped children have repeatedly indicated that help with the pragmatic issues of daily living is their greatest need. When the clinician offers therapy instead of or before help in locating and obtaining financial resources, babysitters, respite care, and information about handling handicap-related sequelae, the family is not likely to view the clinician's help as very useful.

The therapist who can help the family gain the information and child care services that they need may be able to avoid turning these families into patients and, therefore, provide a more positive family-professional experience. Thus, it is essential for therapists who work with any family that has a young handicapped child to build strong collaborative relationships with special educators and other child development specialists.

REFERENCES

Aponte, H. (1976). The family-school interview. *Family Process, 15*, 303–310.

Beavers, J., Hampson, R., Hulgus, Y., & Beavers, R. (1986). Coping in families with a retarded child. *Family Process, 25*, 365–378.

Beckman, P. (1983). Characteristics of handicapped infants: A study of the relationship between child characteristics and stress as reported by mothers. *American Journal of Mental Deficiency, 88*, 150–156.

Beckman-Bell, P. (1981). Child-related stress in families of handicapped children. *Topics in Early Childhood Special Education, 1*(3), 45–53.

Berger, M. (1984). Special education programs. In M. Berger & G.J. Jurkovic (Eds.), *Practicing family therapy in diverse settings* (pp. 142–179). San Francisco: Jossey-Bass.

Berger, M., & Foster, M. (1986). Applications of family therapy theory to research and interventions with families with mentally retarded children. In J.J. Gallagher & P.M. Vietze (Eds.), *Families of handicapped persons: Research, programs and policy issues*. Baltimore: Paul H. Brooks.

Bristol, M.M. (1984). Family resources and successful adaptation to autistic children. In E. Schopler & G. Mesibov (Eds.), *Families of autistic children* (pp. 289–310). New York: Plenum Press.

Bristol, M.M. (in press). Issues in the assessment of single-parent families of young handicapped children. *Journal of the Division of Early Childhood*.

Bristol, M.M., Reichle, N.C., & Thomas, D.D. (1986). *Changing demographics of the American family: Implications for single parent families of handicapped children*. Manuscript submitted for publication.

Bristol, M.M., Schopler, E., & McConnaughey, R. (December 1984). *The prevalence of separation and divorce in unserved families of young autistic and autistic-like children*. Paper presented at the Annual Conference of the Handicapped Children's Early Education Program/Division for Early Childhood, Washington, DC.

Broman, S.H., Nichols, P.L., & Kennedy, W.A. (1975). *Preschool IQ: Prenatal and early developmental correlates*. Hillsdale, NJ: Lawrence Erlbaum Associates.

Farber, B. (1968). *Mental retardation: Its social context and its social consequences*. Boston: Houghton Mifflin.

Foster, M., Berger, M., & McLean, M. (1981). Rethinking a good idea: A reassessment of parent involvement. *Topics in Early Childhood Special Education, 1*, 55–65.

Gallagher, J.J., Scharfman, W., & Bristol, M.M. (1984). The division of responsibilities in families with preschool handicapped and nonhandicapped children. *Journal of the Division for Early Childhood, 8*, 3–11.

Goffman, E. (1963). *Stigma: Notes on the management of spoiled identity*. Englewood Cliffs, NJ: Prentice-Hall.

Greenspan, S.I. (1986). Psychopathology and preventive intervention in infancy: A clinical developmental research approach. In D.C. Farran & J.D. McKinney (Eds.), *Risk in intellectual and psychosocial development* (pp. 129–166). New York: Academic Press.

Harris, S. (1984). Intervention planning for the family of the autistic child: A multilevel assessment of the family system. *Journal of Marital and Family Therapy, 10*, 157–166.

Holroyd, J. (1974). The questionnaire on resources and stress: An instrument to measure family response to a handicapped member. *Journal of the Division for Early Childhood, 6*, 3–13.

Holroyd, J., & McArthur, D. (1976). Mental retardation and stress on the parents: A comparison between Down's syndrome and autism. *American Journal of Mental Deficiency, 80*, 431–436.

Jones, C.W. (1986). *Social networks and adjustment among black, low-income, single-parent families with a retarded child*. Unpublished doctoral dissertation, Georgia State University, Atlanta.

Kazak, A., & Marvin, R. (1984). Differences, difficulties, and adaptation: Stress and social networks in families with a handicapped child. *Family Relations, 33*, 67–77.

Keeney, B.P. (1983). Ecological assessment. In J.C. Hansen & B.P. Keeney (Eds.), *Diagnosis and assessment in family therapy*. Rockville, MD: Aspen Publishers.

Minuchin, S., Rosman, B., & Baker, L. (1978). *Psychosomatic families*. Cambridge, MA: Harvard University Press.

Moses, K.L. (1983). The impact of initial diagnosis: Mobilizing family resources. In J. Mulick & S. Pueschel (Eds.), *Parent-professional partnerships in developmental disability services* (pp. 11–32). Cambridge, MA: Academic Guild Press.

Salzinger, S., Kaplan, S., & Artemyeff, C. (1983). Mothers' personal networks and child maltreatment. *Journal of Abnormal Psychology, 92*, 68–76.

Tew, B., & Laurence, K. (1975). Some sources of stress found in mothers of spina bifida children. *British Journal Preview of Social Medicine, 29*, 27–30.

Turnbull, S.P., & Turnbull, H.R. (1978). *Parents speak out: Views from the other side of the two-way mirror*. Columbus, OH: Charles E. Merril.

Wahler, R.G. (1980). Parent insularity as a determinant of generalization success in family treatment. In S. Salzinger, J. Antrobus, & J. Glick (Eds.), *The ecosystem of the "sick" child* (pp. 187–199). New York: Academic Press.

Wolfensberger, W. (1967). Counseling parents of the retarded. In A. Baumeister (Ed.), *Mental retardation: Appraisal, education, and rehabilitation* (pp. 329–400). Chicago: Aldine.

8. Father-Custody Families: Therapeutic Goals and Strategies

Richard A. Warshak, PhD
Private Practice
and
Clinical Assistant Professor
University of Texas Health Science Center
Dallas, Texas

A lthough psychotherapists have often focused on divorced families, they have for the most part ignored families in which the father has child custody. With more than 1 million children now living with their fathers after the divorce of their parents, however, attention to this population is long overdue.

Father-custody families face many of the same disruptions and challenges that mother-custody families face. Following the dissolution of the nuclear family, the family's basic task is to establish a new stable organization that will facilitate the continued growth and development of family members. At the same time, because father custody after divorce is unconventional in the contemporary United States, the circumstances of father-custody families differ in some important ways from those of mother-custody families. In the past decade, empirical research on father custody has contributed to an understanding of these circumstances (for a review of this literature, see Warshak, 1986). This understanding provides a structure and direction in which to work clinically with father-custody families.

CHARACTERISTICS OF FATHER-CUSTODY FAMILIES

In most families, the initial breakup of a marriage sends a shock wave with reverberations that are felt by everyone in the family for many months,

---

Note: The discussion is limited to families formed as a result of divorce, and does not include father-custody families formed as a result of the mother's death. Although similarities exist between the two types of families, there are also important differences.

sometimes many years. Disruptions occur in intrapsychic and interpersonal realms, as well as in nonpsychological areas, such as housework and employment. A search for effective and stable coping strategies follows a general period of distress. This reaction is similar in both father-custody and mother-custody families.

Children in Father-Custody Homes

The similarities between mother-custody and father-custody families are most apparent in the children's reactions to the separation and their attitudes about the divorce. Regardless of which parent has custody, preadolescent children exhibit common symptoms of stress immediately following the separation. Such symptoms include increased demands for parental attention, fears of abandonment and separation, generalized anxiety, and anger (Bartz & Witcher, 1978; Hetherington, Cox, & Cox, 1982; Wallerstein & Kelly, 1980; Warshak & Santrock, 1983a).

Parents may view the divorce as a solution to their marital problems, but the majority of their children view the *divorce* as the problem. In one study, more than two-thirds of the children in both father-custody homes and mother-custody homes said that they would like their family to be the way it was before the divorce (Warshak & Santrock, 1983b). Interestingly, an average of 3 years had passed since the parents of these children had initially separated. A desire for reconciliation was almost universal, but many fathers and mothers were not consciously aware of their child's wishes for their reconciliation. Most of the children in each group enjoyed their contacts with their non-custodial parent, but more than one-half found the extent of contact inadequate.

There is a popular notion that many children blame themselves for their parents' divorce. Research findings are inconsistent on this point, however, suggesting that clinicians should not be too quick to make such an interpretation (Warshak & Santrock, 1983b; Young, 1983).

> Mr. and Mrs. A. (all names have been changed to protect privacy) requested a consultation in order to evaluate how their daughter, 7-year-old Chloe, was coping with their divorce and to prevent the development of any problems. Midway into the first session with Chloe, the therapist decided to introduce the topic of self-blame.
>
> Therapist: Some boys and girls worry that something *they* did . . .
>
> Chloe: *(interrupting with a tone of annoyance):* I know the divorce wasn't my fault. Why does everyone think that I blame myself for the divorce?
>
> Therapist: Oh, do they?

Chloe: Well, my mother told me it wasn't my fault, my father told me it wasn't my fault, my grandmother and grandpa told me it wasn't my fault, and my teacher told me it wasn't my fault. I never even thought it *was* my fault.

Although some clinicians may think, "The lady doth protest too much," an equally plausible interpretation is that the adults have overdone the reassurances, a not uncommon practice among divorcing parents who want to assuage their guilt.

Fathers with Custody

Immediately after the separation, when children are highly distressed and most in need of high-quality parenting, they often encounter distressed parents who are unable to respond as effectively as usual to their needs. Fathers with custody do not escape the range of negative feelings (e.g., anger, guilt, anxiety, and depression) that are the lot of most divorced spouses. Divorce entails less disruption to a father's self-concept and self-esteem when he maintains custody, however. In fact, his identity as a parent is strengthened, and his relationship with his children is not subject to the constraints of a visiting schedule. Also, as a group, father-custody families are more financially secure than are mother-custody families.

Custodial fathers echo the complaint of custodial mothers that their lives are overburdened. In addition to the demands of their occupation, they must assume single-handedly the household and child care responsibilities usually shared by two parents. The father of a 4-year-old conveyed the weariness of most custodial parents:

There's lots of times when it feels like a big burden, it really does. . . . It's just a lot of work. Everything I do by myself. It seems as if the enormity of the task of arranging things becomes magnified greatly. (Richards & Goldenberg, 1986, p. 157)

Like custodial mothers, custodial fathers find it difficult to coordinate all these responsibilities with a social life. A sense of social isolation and loneliness is paramount, especially among men who had been extremely dependent on their wives for emotional and social support (Luepnitz, 1982).

Family Interaction

In the period immediately following the separation and divorce, child-parent relationships are generally fraught with tension and conflict. The combination of severe emotional stress, job demands, household tasks, child care responsibilities, and dating reduces the time and attention that the custodial parent has available for the children. The diminished parenting heightens the children's sense of deprivation and fuels their anxiety, demands, and anger, which in turn creates more stress for the parent. Guilt over the divorce leads many parents to relax their enforcement of the limits they set, but custodial fathers seem to avoid the discipline problems so commonly experienced by custodial mothers. This may be attributed to the fact that, although custodial fathers become more lenient after the divorce, they are less permissive and less likely to allow their children to control them than are custodial mothers (Luepnitz, 1982; Santrock, Warshak, & Elliott, 1982).

Father-custody families exist in a culture in which it is assumed that child-rearing is women's work and that men are not suited to this task. This belief is reflected in the small proportion of divorced families in which the father retains custody of the children—approximately 1 in 10. As a result of gender role stereotypes, men are *not* socialized to respond to children's emotional needs. Television and films that depict bungling men as helpless in the face of child care tasks create sympathy for custodial fathers and lead to many unsolicited offers of aid (Meredith, 1985). Some custodial fathers themselves express doubt about their abilities in this area. Fiction comes closer to reality in films such as *Kramer vs. Kramer* and *Three Men and a Cradle*. In those portrayals, initially inept men gradually learn to be effective full-time parents and, in the process, develop deep nurturant bonds with their children. Beginning with a peripheral involvement, they gradually make their children's welfare their top priority. Nevertheless, over time fathers are able to acquire these skills.

In two studies, when family interaction was compared in father-custody and mother-custody homes, no differences were observed in the quality of affective involvement that could be attributed to custodial status alone (Luepnitz, 1982; Santrock & Warshak, 1979). Also, after an assessment of a wide range of features of psychological development in seven investigations, not one significant difference was found between children in father-custody homes and those in mother-custody homes that could be attributed to the sex of the custodial parent alone, independent of other factors (Warshak, 1986). (These results do not necessarily apply to preschoolers in father-custody families; there have been no systematic studies of this population.) These findings bear emphasis. They provide no support for the prevailing cultural and judicial preference for mother custody and, thus, challenge the traditions of the past 60 years.

Unique Problems of Father-Custody Families

Father-custody families face certain unique problems because of their atypical status in our culture. They exist in a climate of prejudice, social disapproval, or, at best, wariness and this creates difficulties in several domains. Many people openly express doubts about the father's ability to perform adequately as a single parent. Teachers are apt to suspect physical or psychological illness in father-custody children.

> One father repeatedly took his son to the pediatrician because the boy's teacher thought he was ill. When the teacher remained unconvinced that the child was well, the father asked the physician to report directly to the school that the child was in good health and growing properly. It was only then that the teacher stopped complaining to the father about his son's health (Berry, 1981).

Children in father-custody families find that their friends' parents will not allow their children, particularly their daughters, to spend the night in a home where no mother is present.

In the workplace, custodial fathers encounter unsupportive attitudes from supervisors and co-workers. Employers expect men to regard their job as their top priority; they have little tolerance for a father who must juggle work and child care responsibilities.

> In a job interview, one father emphasized his inability to work past 5 o'clock because he had to pick up his children from day care. During his first week on the job, his employer asked him to stay later; when he explained why he could not stay, he lost his job. It appeared that his employer was so unaccustomed to the idea of a father with primary child care responsibility that he had not taken the father seriously during the job interview.

Men who refuse to work overtime because of their child care responsibilities are perceived as less valuable employees and suffer reduced opportunities for advancement.

Co-workers may be highly critical of a father whose child care duties become evident in the workplace (e.g., by a departure from work to retrieve a sick child from school). Although the criticism may be couched in terms of the inconvenience to the job, there is often a psychodynamic element. The high priority that custodial fathers assign to their children sometimes evokes anxiety in other fathers because of their ambivalence about their own reduced involvement with their children, particularly if these other fathers are divorced; criticizing the custodial father is an effort to ward off guilt and anxiety. Female co-workers with traditional attitudes about gender roles or divorced women whose ex-husbands have threatened or actually initiated challenges to the custody of their children often resent fathers with custody and have a psycho-logical stake in proving that the father-custody life style is not viable. These dynamics also operate with some attorneys and therapists who discourage divorced fathers from seeking more access to their children.

The worse criticisms of father-custody families are borne by noncustodial mothers. These women are social outcasts; they must endure a constant barrage of accusations and the disapproval of their family, friends, and even strangers (Constantatos, 1984; Fischer, 1983; Paskowicz, 1982). Condemned by society, these women must be very clear about their own identities and reasons for not retaining custody, or they will live under a cloud of guilt and self-doubt that is likely to prevent them from having effective and rewarding relationships with their children and may cause them to withdraw from parental involvement.

In clinical settings, noncustodial mothers may blame their problems on society's disapprobation, but the underlying issue is one of self-acceptance. Once they have been helped to accept themselves and their situation, they are able to withstand external criticisms without undue anxiety or guilt. A therapist can make a significant contribution to a father-custody family in this area, because the mother's improved self-esteem will have positive repercussions throughout the family system.

FACTORS MEDIATING THE ADJUSTMENT OF FATHER-CUSTODY FAMILIES

By no means are father-custody families a homogeneous group. They vary in several areas that pose advantages or risks to their adjustment. Among others are: (1) the history of the custody decision, (2) child characteristics, (3) parent characteristics, and (4) support systems.

The Custody Decision

Process of Custody Acquisition. How, why, and when a father acquires custody of his children all affect the family's postdivorce adjustment. Both parents may agree on the arrangement; the mother may unilaterally decide to opt out of full-time parenting, forcing the father to assume custody by default, or there may be threatened or actual litigation for custody. Each of these routes to custody is associated with a different outcome.

Parents who agree on father custody usually have a more cooperative and less conflictual co-parenting relationship. The father feels more in control of his situation, is more prepared to assume household and child care responsibilities, and adjusts more easily to the divorce (Gasser & Taylor, 1976; Mendes, 1976).

When the mother simply decides to relinquish custody, leaving the father no choice, the father is less prepared for his new life situation; moreover, he is usually very anxious and angry about having to assume responsibilities that he neither wanted nor sought. Latent ambivalent feelings about parenthood, denied as long as the mother assumed primary responsibility for child-rearing, may surface. In most of these cases, it was the mother who wanted the divorce, which adds to the father's anger. The level of postdivorce interparental conflict is generally higher in these families than in families that agree on custody. The children are likely to misinterpret their mother's departure and their father's reactions as indications of their worth, rather than as adult problems. This leaves the children more vulnerable to depressive reactions and diminished self-esteem.

When custody is a contested issue and decided in the context of threatened or actual litigation, interparental conflict is highest and may continue indefinitely. These families have the most difficulty adjusting to divorce (Hauser, 1985; Johnston, Campbell, & Tall, 1985).

Reasons for Custody Acquisition. It is important to examine the reasons for the father having custody. The most favorable circumstance occurs when the father retains custody because he is capable of optimally meeting the children's needs. When the mother is psychologically or physically unable to care for the children and the father retains custody by default, the children's postdivorce adjustment is apt to be compromised. For one reason, the father may not be particularly skilled as a parent himself; for another, there is a greater likelihood of earlier deprivation (i.e., abuse or neglect) if an inadequate mother has been primarily responsible for the children. If the divorce results in more consistent and competent parenting, as well as a separation from an abusive mother, the children may experience considerable relief.

Some mothers unilaterally relinquish custody because they have become dissatisfied with the primary care-giver role and want to pursue their career or social life more actively than would be possible if they had sole custody of their children. Financial realities are also a contributing factor in many of these decisions. Although these mothers may attain greater self-actualization and more enjoyment in their relationship with their children, they generally remain conflicted over their custody decision. This may be traced, in part, to their status as social outcasts. In addition, they are more lonely, miss their children, and long for a greater influence over their children's lives (Constantatos, 1984). Such feelings parallel those of most noncustodial fathers.

Father custody is sometimes the result of a child's expressed preference, although the child often feels guilty about favoring one parent. If the child chooses to stay with the father in order to remain in the same neighborhood and school, the decision is usually more palatable to the mother. If the child chooses to live with the father in order to avoid conflicts with the mother, father custody is often less satisfactory to both the parents and their child; it does not usually resolve the conflicts, although it may provide temporary relief to the mother, child, and siblings. If the preference reflects primarily a wish to seek or retain a relationship with the father, the mother is apt to experience a great deal of sadness, guilt, anger, and humiliation. Most mothers take such an expression of preference as a public statement of their inadequacy as a parent.

The least favorable circumstance under which a father acquires custody occurs when the father has no real interest in raising the children, but hopes to use custody as a means to other ends. His goal may be to avoid child support payments, to hurt his ex-wife, or to maintain a more involved relationship with her. The children almost always suffer under such an arrangement, and the level of postdivorce conflict remains high.

Timing of Custody Acquisition. Children may live with their father immediately after the separation; they may live initially with their mother and then, for a variety of reasons, move in with their father; or they may be involved in multiple transfers back and forth, what can be called fluctuating custody arrangement. All things being equal, there are generally fewer problems when the father-custody arrangement begins immediately. Some couples decide at the time of the divorce to transfer custody to the father at a specified future date in order to ensure the continuation of the father-child relationship. This type of planned transfer requires a period of adjustment for all parties, but it usually causes less anguish and conflict than do unanticipated changes in custody.

Adjustment difficulties typically accompany unplanned transfers of custody. Such transfers may occur as a result of intense mother-child conflict or stepfather-child conflict. They may be necessary because the mother is relocating her home, or they may be provoked by a father's anger at his ex-wife's new relationship with another man.

Child Characteristics

Sex. As noted earlier, children in father-custody homes fare just as well as do those in mother-custody homes. Important differences between the adjustment of children in father-custody homes and that of children in mother-custody homes become evident when the sex of the child is taken into account. A consensus of research findings indicates more favorable outcomes for boys in father-custody homes and girls in mother-custody homes (Warshak, 1986). In general, girls in father-custody homes were more anxious, had lower self-esteem, were less mature, and were less likely to be pleased with the custody arrangement. Therefore, the child's sex should be one factor, among many, to be considered in predicting postdivorce functioning.

There are several explanations for the sex-linked pattern of adjustment. A girl's identification with her mother is strained when she lives with her father after divorce, partly because her mother is less available. There is another factor that may be more significant, however. Divorced parents usually devalue their ex-spouse. They convey this attitude to their children either unconsciously or, often, consciously. Moreover, they subtly—or sometimes not so subtly—encourage the children to adopt these negative attitudes themselves, which requires the children to renounce their identifications with the noncustodial parent. As these identifications are a crucial part of a child's self, the children are devaluing central aspects of themselves when they renounce the non-custodial parent. Hence, the low self-esteem that many children of divorce suffer.

In father-custody homes, this effect is more prominent in girls. Although identifications with the opposite sex parent are important for rich personality formation, the most salient identifications are with the same sex parent. The process by which a girl who lives in a father-custody home disowns aspects of her identification with her mother threatens her primary identification as female. The same considerations apply to boys in mother-custody homes.

Identification between parents and children is a two-way street. Parents may interact more effectively and feel more comfortable with a child of the same sex, which may contribute to the better adjustment of children who live with the same sex parent. Most fathers feel that they have less to offer their daughters, and most mothers feel the same about sons.

Some opposite sex custodial parents treat their children as a quasi-spouse. Feeling lonely, emotionally deprived, and stressed, the parent leans on the child for companionship, nurturance, and comfort. Most children are not capable of meeting their parent's emotional needs on a regular basis without sacrificing their own developmental progress, however. The parent, then, is disappointed, and the child is left feeling overwhelmed and inadequate. Child-parent role reversals and emotionally enmeshed families are common outcomes. There is another manner in which children are treated as quasi-spouse. At times, a custodial parent may displace anger at the ex-spouse onto a child who reminds the parent of the ex-spouse. For example, a divorced father may complain contemptuously that his daughter is acting just like her mother. Although these dynamics can operate between parents and children of either sex, most often they are found between mothers and sons or between fathers and daughters.

Treating the child as a quasi-spouse leads to more strain in child-parent relationships and diminishes children's self-esteem, because the children come to see themselves as a source of frustration to their parents. As adults, these children may have to contend with a deep-seated conviction that they cannot meet the expectations of the opposite sex—a conviction that is bound to interfere with their ability to maintain gratifying heterosexual relationships.

Still another possibility is that girls who live in father-custody homes were more likely to have problems that predated the divorce. The current state of research does not allow a definitive statement about this, but it is clear that girls in father-custody homes are more likely to display problems in their development.

Age. The child's current age and the age at the time of the divorce can be expected to mediate postdivorce adjustment. Although there is a need for more research with father-custody families, work with mother-custody families has already shown that divorce has differential effects on children of different ages (Wallerstein & Kelly, 1980). Most studies have focused on preadolescent children, but the outlook may change for these children when they reach adolescence and young adulthood. In mother-custody homes, for example, girls generally cope well with divorce; later in life, however, they display more anxiety and less self-confidence in heterosexual relationships. There is not enough information on father-custody adolescent boys to determine if they evidence parallel problems.

However, there is research indicating that adolescent boys in father-custody homes are less likely to be delinquent and fare no worse than do adolescent boys in mother-custody homes, according to self-report scales of anxiety, sex role development, and self-esteem (Gregory, 1965; Rholes, Clark, & Morgan, 1982). If they have positive involvements with the opposite sex in their younger years, father-custody boys have an advantage over mother-custody girls. Boys have more opportunities for contact with women other than their mother, because most elementary schoolteachers and substitute care-givers are women.

Special Problems. Children in father-custody homes who have problems that predate their parents' divorce have more difficulty coping with the divorce than do those children whose development had been proceeding unhampered. Moreover, problems that had gone unnoticed previous to the divorce (e.g., learning disabilities, attention deficit disorders, and separation anxiety disorders) become evident as the added stress of the divorce overtaxes the children's coping abilities. These children present a more complicated clinical picture, and it is a common error for clinicians to treat the new symptoms merely as reactions to the divorce and to overlook other contributory factors.

Children who have difficult temperaments (Chess & Thomas, 1984) and have always required more time and preparation to accept change do not find it easy to cope with divorce and father custody. Visits with their mother are especially difficult for them. Because consistency in parental behaviors is an essential element in managing a child's difficult temperament, a good co-parenting relationship may be imperative for such a child.

Parent Characteristics

The personality dynamics and emotional status of the parents, including their experiences in their family of origin (e.g., their internal representations of their parents, their relationship to their parents, and their parents' marital relationship), can be expected to influence the functioning of father-custody families. Most therapists are aware of the importance of these factors, but there have been no systematic investigations along these lines.

Co-parenting Relationship. The greater the cooperation and the fewer the conflicts between divorced parents, the more successful the adjustment to the divorce in children from both father-custody and mother-custody homes (Hetherington, Cox, & Cox, 1982; Luepnitz, 1982; Rosen, 1979; Wallerstein & Kelly, 1980). A good co-parenting relationship promotes the children's sense of security, eases the painful loyalty conflicts often engendered in them by the divorce, and allows them to retain and acknowledge their positive feelings for both parents.

Parenting Skills of Fathers. Custodial fathers who are authoritative in their parenting are more likely to raise socially competent children than are fathers who are either overly permissive or excessively harsh and punitive. Authoritative parenting entails setting clear limits and exercising firm control, coupled with warm, attentive involvement and extensive verbal give-and-take. This parenting strategy has been associated with higher levels of self-esteem, maturity, and social responsibility in children from father-custody, mother-custody, and intact families (Baumrind, 1971; Hetherington, Cox, & Cox, 1982; Santrock & Warshak, 1979).

There is a developmental risk when a parent partially transfers the burden of single parenthood to the children. The parent may, for example, delegate to the children responsibility for household chores and care of themselves and younger siblings that far exceeds the children's capacities. Although some custodial fathers treat their children in this fashion, such treatment may be more typical of custodial mothers (Luepnitz, 1982).

Involvement of Mothers. A good relationship with the noncustodial parent can be a major support to children whose parents have divorced. The maintenance of this relationship not only reduces the children's fears of abandonment and loss of love, but also confirms their lack of involvement in their parents' disputes. In mother-custody families, continuing contact between the children and their noncustodial father plays an important role in the successful adjustment of the children, particularly the boys (Hess & Camara, 1979; Hetherington, Cox, & Cox, 1982; Kurdek & Berg, 1983; Wallerstein & Kelly, 1980). In father-custody families, the effect of the mother's visiting relationship on the children's adjustment has not been extensively studied, but there is reason to believe that the pattern resembles that in mother-custody families.

Children and adults who were raised in father-custody homes are less likely to look back on the divorce as traumatic when they have had frequent access to their mother (Rosen, 1977). Furthermore, girls who have a positive relationship with their noncustodial mother are more likely to display competence in their peer relationships (Camara, 1982).

Support Systems

Children in divorced families more often receive substitute care than their counterparts in intact families. Although there are no consistent findings regarding the difference between father-custody families and mother-custody families in this matter, substitute child care has been linked to healthier functioning in both types of families (Luepnitz, 1982; Santrock & Warshak, 1979). There are several plausible explanations for this association.

It is likely that the availability of substitute child care makes it possible for children to receive a greater amount and a higher quality of adult attention, both from the additional care-givers and from the custodial parent (because the parent's emotional resources are less depleted). On the other hand, because children who are better adjusted are more pleasant to be around, the parents may receive more offers of substitute child care (e.g., from relatives) or may be more likely to entrust their children to the care of other adults. It is also possible that both the availability of support systems and the associated positive adjustment of the children reflect the social competence of the custodial parent. Parents who do not obtain external support may be more isolated, more depressed, and less able to respond appropriately to their children's needs.

Relatives and friends who understand and accept the father-custody arrangement can provide important support to both parents by sanctioning their unconventional family structure. Unfortunately, as discussed earlier, custodial fathers and noncustodial mothers often face severe criticisms.

THERAPEUTIC INTERVENTIONS: GOALS AND STRATEGIES

During the early phases of divorce, therapists can make significant clinical contributions, such as advising the parents on custody issues, promoting co-parenting relationships, and preparing the children for the separation. Then therapists can help to improve parent-child relationships and strengthen support systems.

Intervening in the Early Phases of Divorce

Ideally, therapeutic work with father-custody families begins before the new family structure is formed. When families consult a therapist before the separation, the therapist is in a unique position to help prevent problems. Moreover, clinicians are often called upon to assist parents and courts in determining optimal custody and visitation arrangements. In the past, one standard was the basis for such recommendations: the mother's "fitness." Only if the mother were grossly negligent or abusive would clinicians recommend against mother custody.

Unfortunately, many mental health care professionals continue to base their recommendations on this standard, even though there is no evidence to support this position. Custodial fathers *can* raise their children competently, and many are doing so as effectively as custodial mothers. Thus, in custody consultations and evaluations, clinicians should consider an array of factors that affect postdivorce functioning:

- the quality of interaction between father and child, and between mother and child
- the parenting styles and coping abilities of each parent
- the amount of time each will be able to spend with the children
- the degree to which each parent will facilitate the child's relationship with the other
- the availability of support systems

Characteristics of the children such as their age, personality, and special needs are also relevant. Finally, research findings suggest that some weight should be assigned to the child's sex in any effort to predict the outcome of different living arrangements.

Most couples who have decided to divorce expect that the mother will retain custody of the children and the father will see the children 4 days per month. They rarely entertain alternatives to this arrangement. By underscoring the crucial importance of the children's access to *both* parents, clinicians can expand the range of options available to the family. This may lead to more father-custody and joint custody agreements.

Many noncustodial parents discount or are unaware of their continuing importance in their children's lives. Some are concerned that frequent contact with their children will give them a sense of insecurity or fuel their fantasies of reconciliation. These misconceptions may result in an insufficient quantity and quality of contact between noncustodial parents and their children. Once established, this pattern is difficult to change. Therefore, it is essential to address this issue during a predivorce consultation. It is surprising how often a brief intervention at this time has a long-term positive effect on the non-custodial parent–child relationship.

Promoting a Cooperative Co-parenting Relationship. In working with separating couples, the therapist must remember that the behavior observed at the predivorce consultation is likely to change in the near future. When the consultation occurs shortly after the decision to divorce, some couples present themselves as "model divorcing spouses," each eager to support the other's continuing involvement with their children. Most are unprepared for the intensity of the rage that they will experience as part of the adjustment process; however, the clinician's failure to anticipate this rage can counteract the efficacy of interventions designed to promote a co-parenting alliance.

> Mrs. B. announced to her husband that she was leaving him and that, in her opinion, their two children should stay with him. Mr. B. dealt with his feelings in his characteristic stoic manner, saying little, while his sad eyes and clenched jaw spoke volumes. The couple consulted a therapist for advice on helping their children adjust to their new living arrangement. The therapist underscored the importance of Mrs. B.'s continued active involvement with the children. Still stunned by the blow of the impending separation, Mr. B. pledged his support.
>
> Two weeks later, Mrs. B. agreed to stay with the children one morning so that Mr. B. could leave early for work. She was late arriving at the home, which caused Mr. B. to be late for work. After that time, Mr. B. refused to allow Mrs. B. to see the children beyond the strict terms of their divorce decree, ostensibly to protect the children from the feelings of insecurity that they would experience as a result of their mother's "inconsistency." Mr. B., convinced that his decision was guided solely by consideration of the children's best interests, would not agree to explore with the therapist the dynamics, logic, or destructive impact of his decision.

Clearly, therapeutic strategies in predivorce interventions must go beyond the essential education and advice. An effective technique is to anticipate and discuss with parents the probable emergence of rage and the possible manifestation of rage in behaviors that are detrimental to the children's welfare. The following monologue is an example.

> Your children are fortunate to have parents who are determined not to let the divorce interfere with their need for their mother and father. In the coming weeks and months, however, you may find yourself thinking of reasons to interfere with your children's access to each other. Perhaps the children will cry or misbehave each time they go from one home to the other. This is a common reaction to the stress of change and separation from a loved parent. It should not automatically be taken as proof that the children are suffering by being with the other parent.
>
> Unfortunately, some parents will seize upon any excuse to justify keeping their ex-spouse from the children. If you are perceptive, you will realize that any wish you have to keep the children from your ex-spouse really comes from your anger and your wish to punish your ex; it has little to do with what is best for the children.
>
> When you pay close attention to your children they will constantly remind you that no matter how much you may try to justify your behavior, no matter how much you may hate each other, your children want and need *both* of you. Your excuses may help you feel better about your behavior temporarily, but deep down you will feel uneasy because you can't escape the knowledge that you are indulging your wishes for retaliation at your children's expense. This will backfire because, in hurting your children, you will be hurting your relationship with them. Your children may hold it against you. Furthermore, children who have inadequate contact with one of their parents are more likely to develop emotional problems, and a disturbed child is much more difficult to raise. Wise parents recognize residual angry feelings toward the former spouse as natural without having to act on them.

The aim of this intervention is to enlist parents in a therapeutic alliance to defuse potentially destructive behavior. It serves three purposes:

1. It prepares the parents to recognize the rage when it emerges, despite its many disguises.
2. It encourages the parents to maintain a conscious awareness of the destructive impact of any interference in their children's relationship with the other parent.

3. It links the parents' self-esteem as parents to their ability to facilitate their children's relationship with their former spouse.

An intervention like this preempts the effective use of rationalizations by revealing, in advance, the hidden motive (i.e., the wish to punish the ex-spouse by obstructing access to the children). When they understand that such actions are harmful to the children, few loving parents can use their children in this manner. Parents who subsequently resort to these maneuvers, despite such intervention, are usually struggling with overwhelming rage and significant ego deficits.

Predivorce interventions usually take place at a time of great stress. Because stress tends to disrupt cognitive operations, it is important to phrase therapeutic communications in a manner that will facilitate processing and recall. For example, it may be necessary to repeat significant messages several times. In addition, it may be helpful to be concrete and graphic about possible adverse outcomes for the children, as this increases the motivational impact of the communication. Clinicians should determine what is likely to "touch the parent's button" in this regard. For some parents, it is a future of gross academic underachievement; for others, it is the prospect of chronic encopresis.

Helping Parents Prepare Their Children. It is surprising how often parents fail to tell their children why they are divorcing or to explain the family's new living arrangements. When parents do not talk openly about such matters, the children are less likely to voice their own concerns. Instead, the children will develop a variety of fantasies that explain the divorce and custody situation, none of which may correspond in the least with reality.

If the father-custody disposition results from the mother's need for autonomy and liberation from full-time mothering, it is necessary to assure the children that the decision does not reflect the children's worth, but their mother's needs. This is a very difficult concept for children to grasp. Children who see little of their noncustodial parent invariably suffer a loss of self-esteem, with or without treatment. Nevertheless, the therapist should try to help the children appreciate and internalize this communication, on a conscious and unconscious level, and to seek substitute gratification (for example, spending more time with friends, older siblings, and grandparents).

When helping parents prepare their children for the separation, therapists should be alert to the parents' feelings about the breakup, as they will potentially color the announcement to the children.

Mr. & Mrs. C. met with a therapist shortly after they decided to end their marriage. They were seeking assistance in working out custody arrangements, but their immediate objective was to determine the best way to tell their child about the divorce.

The therapist asked Mr. C., who had requested the divorce, what he thought he might say to his son. In reply, Mr. C. launched into a recitation that emphasized all the positive aspects of the breakup. The therapist commented that, if the parent seeking the divorce were to err in informing the children about the divorce, it was likely to be in the direction of minimizing the traumatic nature of the breakup. Mr. C. was able to see that this, in fact, was what he had planned to do. He then acknowledged his guilt and his fear of emotionally harming his son.

This discussion made it easier for Mr. C. to accept the possibility that his guilt could keep him from allowing his son to express sad, anxious, and angry feelings as a first step in the grieving process. When the parents subsequently broke the news to their son, Mr. C. was able to temper his optimism by recalling the discussion with the therapist.

When children learn about their parents' impending divorce, many begin acting, consciously and unconsciously, in ways designed to bring about a reconciliation. Parents may need help to recognize the underlying meaning of this behavior.

Seven-year-old Suzie D., in the temporary custody of her father, kept "accidentally" tearing her dresses and then advising her father to "call Mommy and tell her. She'll come over and sew them." Although the latent motive of this ploy seems obvious, Suzie's parents did not recognize her intent to reunite them. Blinded by their anger at each other and the stress of separation, each blamed the other for Suzie's problem. Suzie's mother assumed that Mr. D. was not adequately supervising their daughter and considered this confirmation of her suspicions that Mr. D. was unfit for custody. Suzie's father thought that Suzie expected her mother to let her "get away" with destructive behavior and considered it another consequence of Mrs. D.'s overly permissive parenting. This type of misunderstanding kept the parents involved in repetitive litigation around custody and visitation issues.

Co-parenting relationships improve when parents are oriented toward (1) recognizing symptoms of distress in their children and (2) regarding the distress as a mandate to respond jointly to their children's underlying emotional needs.

Facilitating the Mother-Child Relationship

An important goal of therapy with father-custody families is to improve the level and quality of the mother's involvement with her children. This goal involves three subgoals: (1) to ensure an adequate amount of contact between the mother and her children, (2) to assist the mother in managing the children's behavior, and (3) to help the mother overcome the internal and external barriers to fulfillment in her role as noncustodial parent. Clearly, the mother's participation in therapy is a key ingredient in the attainment of these goals.

Unfortunately, many noncustodial mothers are anxious to create a substantial geographical distance between themselves and their ex-husbands. These women are predominantly those who believe that their identities have been stifled in a suffocating marriage. By casting off the roles of wife and full-time mother, they hope to flourish as individuals. In their search for individuation, however, these women confuse the goal of *psychological separateness* with *physical separation*. Therapeutic intervention can help them to realize that true autonomy consists not of changing one's state, but of changing one's state of mind.

When the mother already lives far away from the children and is unable to have frequent contact with them, the therapist can offer suggestions to bridge the gap. For example, the mother may contact her child's teacher and ask to be kept informed of the child's progress through copies of report cards. If the mother sends self-addressed, stamped envelopes, the teacher is more likely to comply with the request.

Some noncustodial mothers hesitate to become involved with their children because they believe that their children no longer value them. Often feeling guilty and depressed, such a mother assumes that her children share her ex-husband's low opinion of her. The therapist should help this mother understand the enduring nature of attachment bonds. Also, it is effective in this situation to encourage the children to assert their desires for more contact with their mother. This is best accomplished in family sessions.

During marriage, many women relied on the authority of their husbands to support their disciplinary measures with their children. When these mothers are on their own, their lack of authority is acutely evident and creates a great deal of tension and conflict in mother-child interactions. In response to the noncompliant behavior of their children, some mothers set too many limits and give too many commands, which the children ignore or resist. Ineffective communication and inconsistent discipline seem to be the order of the day. If the relationship continues to be mutually frustrating, contact between the mother and her children may gradually decline. These mothers can improve their parenting practices by learning to attend more frequently to positive behaviors, increase nurturance, and more consistently enforce limits. Video-taped parent-child interactions can assist them in identifying their ineffective approaches.

Some mothers find that their efforts to control their children's behavior are defeated by their fear of alienating the children. Guilt over leaving the children with their father prompts many noncustodial mothers to adopt an overly permissive parenting style. If the underlying guilt is not addressed, therapeutic efforts may flounder. In fact, helping noncustodial mothers deal with their guilt is a critical issue in therapy with father-custody families. If the guilt of the noncustodial mother remains at a high level, it can be evoked during each contact, and the accompanying anxiety can discourage frequent contact. Once the guilt abates, the possibility of a more gratifying mother-child relationship increases.

A particularly trying circumstance for a mother is when her child asks to live with her father. Often the mother's response to this request is one of hurt and self-blame. Just as the bereaved are plagued by thoughts of what they could have done to prevent a loved one's death, so the mother will blame herself for her child's preference. In part this stems from inadequate understanding of developmental needs, in part it is a defense against anger, and in part the guilt serves the purpose of assuaging feelings of helplessness. Feeling guilty implies that one had some control over the situation; maintaining the belief that she caused the child's preference to live with the father allows the mother to believe that reversing the preference is within her power.

The mother must be helped to appreciate that she has little, if any, control over her child's preference. In most cases the mother's behavior is not a major contributing factor to the child's preference. Rather, when the preference is stated at the outset of the separation, the usual motivation is a desire to maintain consistency of home, neighborhood, school, and friends. When the preference entails a shift in living arrangements, it most likely reflects a developmental need to have a closer relationship with the father. In some cases it may *appear* that a child's decision is a reaction to excessive conflict with mother. However, the conflict itself may be prompted by the child's need to maintain some psychological distance from the mother. For a boy this may be in the service of preserving a strong masculine identification, especially if he is the only male in a female-headed household.

The therapist should help the mother understand her child's preference in terms of these factors and accept the child's needs as different from her own. This is the type of stance that is the sine qua non of parenting adolescents. But as one mother of a ten year old remarked, "I always knew my child would grow up and leave home some day. I just wasn't prepared for it to come so soon. What have I done wrong?" In those instances in which the mother's mistreatment *was* a major factor in the child's decision to live with the father, the mother should be helped to confront and accept her past errors and to do whatever is possible to repair the damage that has been done.

Facilitating the Father-Child Relationship

Two areas in which many custodial fathers need assistance are (1) accepting the custodial arrangements and (2) improving parenting skills. A man who actively sought custody of his children is usually prepared for the attendant responsibilities and has little ambivalence about the custody disposition. In many cases, however, the mother has unilaterally relinquished custody and unexpectedly left the father with primary responsibility for the children's care. In this situation, the father not only faces the challenges of single parenthood, but also must deal with his reactions to having it thrust upon him. Indeed, in order to cope effectively with the demands of his family, a father must come to terms with the reality of the custody arrangement.

> Mr. E. requested a consultation with a therapist at the suggestion of his son's teacher, who was concerned about the boy's non-compliant behavior in preschool. Nine months before the initial interview, after announcing her wish for a separation and her feeling that she could not handle her two children alone, Mrs. E. had moved out of the family home. When therapy began, Mr. E. was unemployed.
>
> In his therapy sessions, Mr. E. complained bitterly about the problems that beset most single custodial fathers. He could not seem to make adequate child care arrangements, and he could not find a position that would accommodate his parental responsibilities. Mr. E. described his dilemmas as though they were insurmountable, but he appeared more angry than depressed about the situation. It seemed to the therapist that Mr. E. was not doing all he could to help himself and his family.
>
> The therapist began to focus on the meaning that his failure to cope well had for Mr. E., and the following picture emerged. Before marrying, Mr. and Mrs. E. had agreed that they would not have children. He had a daughter from his previous marriage and was sure he did not want any more children. After 7 years of marriage, however, Mrs. E. began pressing her desire for children, and her husband agreed. Now, when the children were 4 and 6 years old, she had left him with full responsibility for their care. To make matters worse, Mrs. E. refused to discuss her reasons for leaving and would not agree to participate in any form of conjoint treatment. (Mrs. E. did provide a developmental his-

tory of her son and attended a feedback session in which the therapist offered recommendations. Her mood and affect during these sessions suggested that she was suffering from a moderate-to-severe emotional disturbance, but she did not accept a referral for treatment.)

Mr. E.'s failure to cope was now more understandable. He was exhibiting a passive-aggressive type of defense that the therapist labeled "failing to get back." He was failing to get back (recover) his equilibrium, and by failing, was unconsciously getting back at his wife for leaving him in this unwelcome situation. After sorting out his anger at his wife and his ambivalence about parenthood, Mr. E. was able to accept the reality of the custody disposition and begin the process of effectively reorganizing his life.

Therapy with the E. family illustrates the flexibility needed in structuring sessions. The therapist met with Mr. E. alone in order to explore his resistance to coping; no useful purpose would have been served by allowing the children to learn of their father's parental ambivalence just after they felt abandoned by their mother. When the sessions focused more directly on the father-child relationship, however, the children's presence was an asset. The therapist was able to facilitate better interaction between Mr. E. and his children by such techniques as modeling optimal responses to the children.

The parenting skills in which fathers need the most help are the identification of their children's feelings and effective communication. Fathers of young children can learn to use dolls and play materials to facilitate communication with their children, as is done in play therapy; most parents are surprised and delighted when they discover how children unconsciously project their feelings onto these materials. Reading his children a book about other children's reactions to divorce can sensitize a father to his own children's feelings and, thus, serve as a springboard for further discussion. If the father's parents are divorced (an increasingly common phenomenon), an exploration of his reactions and memories of the experience can help him recognize his children's emotions. In general, the less a father disowns his dependency needs, the better able he will be to recognize and respond to his children's needs for nurturance. It can be helpful to have fathers acknowledge their deficits openly to their children and instruct the children to be vocal about their emotional needs. The children can practice this approach during therapy.

Most fathers respond to their children's expressions of emotions in ways that encourage the children to hide and repudiate their feelings (e.g., by criticizing and lecturing). Therapists can help fathers learn to communicate understanding. Also, custodial fathers must learn to accept behaviors in their children that reflect identifications with their mother, as children cannot renounce these identifications without depreciating themselves.

Strengthening Support Systems

Father-custody families are stressed families. The families that cope best with the stress are those with extraparental supports. Unfortunately, however, the family often loses part of its support system—one set of grandparents—as a consequence of divorce. This is rarely the grandparents' wish; rather, it usually reflects a spillover of conflict from the marital dyad to the extended family that causes the custodial parent to withhold access to the children. This is regrettable because grandparents have an especially important role to play after a separation.

Children's self-esteem benefits enormously when they are able to see themselves as a source of joy to their parents. The parental anxiety and depression that follow a separation deprives their children of this valuable experience. Grandparents who take obvious pleasure in their grandchildren offer a valuable antidote to this deprivation. They can also offer children a needed sense of stability and a haven from the parental hostilities. In order for grandparents to have maximum beneficial impact, they must keep their involvement in the marital turmoil to a minimum. Toward this end, therapists should work to establish an alliance with all the grandparents and help them to assume a supportive role in the postdivorce family structure.

Parents can benefit from participation in adult self-help groups, such as Parents Without Partners and Mothers Without Custody. Children can benefit from any intervention that relieves stress during the postseparation phase. Although parents may feel helpless in reducing divorce-related tensions, they can obtain help for children's problems that may have gone unnoticed previous to the breakup. This help could take the form of organized peer activities, psychotherapy, educational tutoring, or other remedial work.

On a wider scope, mental health professionals can strengthen societal support for father-custody families by working to correct myths that lead to social censure. Cultural biases about the roles that men and women should play in their children's lives have caused pain to mothers who attempted to step out of the bounds of full-time parenting, to fathers who wished to increase their participation in parenting, and to children who found their living arrangements determined more by tradition than by the needs of the family. Although custodial fathers and noncustodial mothers must work through their own ambivalent attitudes about their unconventional roles, there is no doubt that life would be easier for father-custody families if they were accepted more readily by society.

Father-custody families may become more common in the future, but for now, these families are pioneers. Therefore, therapists who work with these families are working largely in uncharted territory. Empirical studies of father-custody families that carry direct implications for clinical intervention are needed. I hope I have succeeded in demonstrating these implications and, in the process, alerting therapists to clinically significant issues and providing useful suggestions for helping families deal with these issues.

REFERENCES

Bartz, K.W., & Witcher, W.C. (1978, Sept.-Oct.). When fathers get custody. *Children Today, 2–5,* 35.

Baumrind, D. (1971). Current patterns of parental authority. *Developmental Psychology Monographs, 4*(1, Part 2), 1–103.

Berry, K.K. (1981). The male single parent. In I.R. Stuart & L.E. Abt (Eds.), *Children of separation and divorce* (pp. 34–53). New York: Van Nostrand Reinhold.

Camara, K.A. (1982, July). *Social interaction of children in divorced and intact households.* Paper presented at the International Congress of Psychiatry and Allied Professions, Dublin, Ireland.

Chess, S., & Thomas, A. (1984). *Origins and evolution of behavior disorders.* New York: Bruner/ Mazel.

Constantatos, M. (1984). *Non-custodial versus custodial divorced mothers: Antecedents and consequences of custody choice.* Unpublished doctoral dissertation, University of Texas Health Science Center at Dallas.

Fischer, J.L. (1983). Mothers living apart from their children: A study in stress and coping. *Alternative Lifestyles, 4*(2), 218–227.

Gasser, R., & Taylor, C. (1976). Role-adjustment of single-parent fathers. *The Family Coordinator, 25,* 397–401.

Gregory, I. (1965). Anterospective data following childhood loss of a parent: I. Delinquency and high school dropout. *Archives of General Psychiatry, 13,* 99–109.

Hauser, B.B. (1985). Custody in dispute: Legal and psychological profiles of contesting families. *Journal of the American Academy of Child Psychiatry, 24,* 575–582.

Hess, R., & Camara, K. (1979). Post-divorce family relationships as mediating factors in the consequences of divorce for children. *Journal of Social Issues, 35*(4), 79–96.

Hetherington, E.M., Cox, M., & Cox, R. (1982). Effects of divorce on parents and children. In M.E. Lamb (Ed.), *Nontraditional families* (pp. 233–288). Hillsdale, NJ: Erlbaum.

Johnston, J.R., Campbell, L.E.G., & Tall, M.C. (1985). Impasses to the resolution of custody and visitation disputes. *American Journal of Orthopsychiatry, 55*(1), 112–129.

Kurdek, L.A., & Berg, B. (1983). Correlates of children's adjustment to their parents' divorces. In L.A. Kurdek (Ed.), *Children and divorce.* San Francisco: Jossey-Bass.

Luepnitz, D.A. (1982). *Child custody.* Lexington, MA: Heath.

Mendes, H. (1976). Single fathers. *The Family Coordinator, 25,* 439–444.

Meredith, D. (1985, June). Dad and the kids. *Psychology Today,* 62–67.

Paskowicz, P. (1982). *Absentee mothers.* New York: Universe Books.

Rholes, W.S., Clark, T.L., & Morgan, R. (1982). *The effects of single father families on personality development.* Unpublished manuscript, Department of Psychology, Texas A & M University, College Station, Texas.

Richards, C.A., & Goldenberg, I. (1986). Fathers with joint physical custody of young children: A preliminary look. *American Journal of Family Therapy, 14,* 154–162.

Rosen, R. (1977). Children of divorce: What they feel about access and other aspects of the divorce experience. *Journal of Clinical Child Psychology, 6,* 24–27.

Rosen, R. (1979). Children of divorce: An evaluation of two common assumptions. *Canadian Journal of Family Law, 2,* 403–415.

Santrock, J.W., & Warshak, R.A. (1979). Father custody and social development in boys and girls. *Journal of Social Issues, 35,* 112–135.

Santrock, J.W., Warshak, R.A., & Elliott, G.L. (1982). Social development and parent-child interaction in father-custody and stepmother families. In M.E. Lamb (Ed.), *Nontraditional families.* Hillsdale, NJ: Erlbaum.

Wallerstein, J.W., & Kelly, J.B. (1980). *Surviving the break-up: How children and parents cope with divorce.* New York: Basic Books.

Warshak, R.A. (1986). Father-custody and child development: A review and analysis of psychological research. *Behavioral Sciences and the Law, 4,* 185–202.

Warshak, R.A., & Santrock, J.W. (1983a). Children of divorce: Impact of custody disposition on social development. In E.J. Callahan & K.A. McCluskey (Eds.), *Life-span developmental psychology* (pp. 289–314). New York: Academic Press.

Warshak, R.A., & Santrock, J.W. (1983b). The impact of divorce in father-custody and mother-custody homes: The child's perspective. In L.A. Kurdek (Ed.), *Children and divorce* (pp. 29–46). San Francisco: Jossey-Bass.

Young, D.M. (1983). Two studies of children of divorce. In L.A. Kurdek (Ed.), *Children of divorce* (pp. 61–70). San Francisco: Jossey-Bass.

Index